The Truth About Calcium

Keys to a
Whole Body Bone Building Lifestyle
&
Osteoporosis Prevention

BY
Catie Wyman-Norris

He is the free man whom the truth makes free,
and all are slaves beside

—Cowper

This book is dedicated to my precious sister Joni,
who was taken way too soon;
and to the many that have needlessly suffered
and even died from osteoporosis and bone loss.

May this book be a bright light to abundant health,
happiness & a stronger body.

And to those industry's that knowingly or otherwise choose
to continue marketing products that keep this "Silent Epidemic" going.
My wish for you is that you will learn from this book and that the
causes you make can and will change to create value
and promote goodness.

First published 2008

First Edition, First Printing, December, 2008

Printed in the United States of America

Cover Design by Patricia Bacall, Bacall:Creative
Composition and interior design by Anne M. Landgraf, Brooklyn BookWorks

Published by:
KD Did, Inc.
(888) 456–1597. Calabasas, CA 91302.

ISBN 0-9801173-2-1

www.energyessentials.com

Contents

Chapter Seven

Acknowledgements

Special thanks to my love, Tony O'Donnell, N.D. who's consistent love and inspiration has been the wind beneath my wings. Thanks for waiting. I love you.

To my children, Ashley & Toren—may you strive to live this books wisdom: continuing to become strong, happy, healthy, conscious human beings. I love you.

To my family, my mother—Lucy, father—Joe, Steve, Nancy, Jimmy, Tom, Peggy, Chris, Joni, Susie, Charlie (Michelle), & Joey. It was our destiny to arise from such a beautiful, bountiful family to create a legacy that will emanate many generations. I love you all so much.

To Brad Norris. Thanks for your support always. May your life's mission bring you happiness and fulfillment.

To Mandy Mawer my right and left arm. You are a precious, sensitive angel in my life. Thank you for all you do.

To Robert & Yolanda Villatoro—Thanks for making our lives so much easier. You are appreciated beyond words.

To Shari Celusta—what a blessing that fate brought us together. I love everything about as do our customers. May the Roar of the Lioness always be in you my friend!!!!

To Lori Gurin. Thank you for your undying efforts in spreading the truth about calcium and real, whole foods. Hugs and bless you always.

To Debi & Steve Wyman. Wow! How wonderful to see you transform your lives and so many others. You are truly dear to our hearts. We love you so much.

Melissa Block—my thanks to you and your wonderful help and research to help make this an outstanding book to help so many.

Thank you Derry Schroer for your help in getting the ball started and bringing life to the research for this book.

To Linda Ory. Bless you for sharing your story and study of how you have helped build your bones by these nutrients at 65 years young! Your story has gone against what the mass marketed information has drilled into us for years. Thank you deeply friend.

To Darbe Nokes. How special your spirit and courage is. I am so sorry your momma had such a painful passing. This book is dedicated to her.

To Noba Jones. How you have suffered from strokes, fractures and multiple health challenges. How sad you were never told of your deficiencies and how to help them. This book is dedicated to you dear lady.

To Melinda & Jason Krupicka. You are family and always will be. I love you much sis & bro! Thanks for your love and support.

To Sharon, Susan, & Kevin from Energy Essentials of Henderson, NV. You have really helped change lives as you have changed your own. I love what you have done and am so proud to have you as friends.

To April Mow, my dear friend. Thanks for your precious love and caring always. I will never forget your kindness dear friend. How special you are to me.

To Susie & Gary Riggs. How precious your family is to us. I think of the pain you have suffered Susie and your great health strides and it continues to give me hope of God's graciousness to bring us together so we can live better, happier lives. I love you both so much.

To Lauren Monroe & Rick Allen. Thank you for your friendship and for your belief in the human spirit to evolve, grow and heal through your wonderful work with Raven Drum. Bless you both.

To Marjorie Rothstein. Bless you for your goodness in helping others and making their lives so beautiful. I love you.

To Beth Miller. Bless you and all the wonderful work you do to help so many suffering. I love you friend.

To Darin Olien. I love what you stand for friend.

To Steve Valiquette. How you care for your friends and fellow team mates health & well being. You are a dear friend. Bless you always.

To Gabby Reece & Laird Hamilton. May you continue to inspire your followers in true health always. Thank you dear friends.

To Roma Downey and Mark Burnett. Your philanthropic work to help the many in Operation Smile get back their smiles has also helped fund the research to help learn of the potential nutritional deficiencies that may be related to Cleft Lip & Pallet malformations (critical research has been included in this book) that so many in malnourished countries suffer from. A percentage from the proceeds of this book will continue to help fund this crucial research. God Bless you both.

To Daryl Hannah. Your vision & values continue to inspire people to do the right thing. Thank you for being real and genuine in your mission & life. This book is printed on recycled paper my friend.

Victor, Ms. Alice & Captain Vic—Thank you for your friendship always. You are family always!

To Bill O'Brien. Your Troubles are Over!!!! Thanks for your friendship and precious support for our work in health. I wish you deep happiness friend.

To Dr's. Mark Anthony, D.C.—may all Doctor's be blessed with your wisdom, passion and desire to truly help heal and change the core of their patients lives. Bless you always!

To Cheryl & Dr. Bob Martin, thanks for your unending love and support for us and for your wonderful radio show that enlightens so many to the truths that need to be told. Your courage gives us all courage.

To the Father of Chelation, Gary Gordon, M.D. Without your truth's, we'd continue to be in darkness and continue to suffer from the mass marketing scandals that take so many lives each and every day! Thank you and your words will greatly impact this devastating epidemic as we get the truth out. Bless you and Alexandra many times over.

To the wonderful stores who believe so deeply in the power of real, whole foods and supplements—bless you always: P.C. Greens (Mike, Lonnie, Victor), Vitamin Barn (Gene, Lucy, Kat, Susan, Freddie, Carlos), The Euphoria Company (Jenabai). Natures Mart (Jacy, Tom, Jackie), Lassen's (Tom, Ann, Amber, Joshua, Janet & Michelle), Healthy Habit Health Foods (Chris, Josh & all), AZ Health (Lisa, Carol, Michael & Roxie, Lyndon, Noah, Marianne, Jerry, Patrick, Gail), Ken at The Family Nutrition Center in Glendale AZ, John at the Vitamin House in Sun City, AZ, A-1 Nutrition (Saleem), all the many Hi-Health Stores (Chris), to all the wonderful Whole Foods Stores and the many others. Thank you all so much.

To Julia & John Churan, your friendship is so dear, precious & refreshing. Thank you for your genuineness dear friends.

To Stacey Jenel Smith, your words touch hearts, entertain, but most importantly share the truth that so often gets swept under the rug. Thank you for all your truths.

To John Anderson of Isagenix International, thank you for your wisdom of nutrition and sharing the strength of the elephants. You are a champion.

To Jael & Nina at Happy Cooking, LTD. Thank you for opening my eyes on the dangers of most cookware and how we can get better nutrition from our foods. Bless you friends.

To Dr. Stacy Olson, D.C. and her amazing staff—you are family and I treasure our friendship much.

To Dr. Reddy, PhD—your understanding and grasp of nourishing and healing through whole foods & herbs has helped so many. Thank you friend & Namaste'

To Dr. John Gray—how inspiring you are to so many! Thanks for being in our lives. We are all better from your wonderful books and wisdom.

To Neal Levitt, Love your entrepreneurial spirit in health. You are always helping people. Blessings Always.

To Dr. Earl Mindell, R.PH, PhD and Gail, Thank you for your friendship and wisdom. You have paved the way to bring real food nutrition back to the people for health. Bless you both.

To Dr. Colin Campbell and your wonderful China Study. Thank you for your humanity and doing the right thing. This study and book will truly change lives and shed the truth of better choices for a healthful life(style). You are truly a great Doctor and human being. Bless you.

Introduction

Americans have gotten the message about calcium and bone health, right? They take calcium supplements. They get their daily servings of dairy. Little do they know that the equation of standard-issue calcium supplements plus plentiful dairy do not add up to strong bones. That they may, in fact, be powerful contributors to bone *loss* . . . and to the general decline in health so many people experience during their 50s and beyond.

Yes, you read it right: people in the United States, who consume more calcium than any other nation, have one of the *highest rates* of osteoporotic-related fractures on the planet. What's more, while our diet contains substantial amounts of calcium from animals (like cheese and milk), statistics demonstrate unequivocally that those who consume the most dairy have the highest rates of osteoporotic fractures. Our rates of osteoporosis far exceed those of people in less developed countries, where dairy is rarely or never eaten.

In an interview with the Beverage Institute, published online at www.beverageinstitute.org, world-renowned calcium researcher Robert Heaney, M.D., stated: "In simple terms, to be healthy, bones need two basic requirements: food and work. As recently as two generations ago, people ate a lot of food—3,000 or 4,000 calories a day—which made them more likely to get needed nutrients. They also walked everywhere and did a lot of physical work. Today, a typical female is sedentary and might eat only 1,400 calories a day, mostly from nutrient-poor foods. So, generally, we're not meeting the basic requirements needed for strong, healthy bones." As a matter of fact, we aren't even getting the nourishment to sustain many basic metabolic life processes. The late Nobel Prize winner, Dr. Albert Szent Gyorgi (1893–1986) said, "Where there are minerals—there is LIFE! Where there are little or no minerals—there is NO LIFE!" As the most abundant mineral in the body, calcium is critical for our bone & teeth formation as well as approximately 350 different metabolic processes. Without calcium and the 17 or so other nutrients to build strong bones, we would crumble—as we are seeing right before our eyes today. This has led to the last two to three generations having serious challenges with bone strength because of poor diet and lack of activity. It is estimated that over half of our population in the United States suffers from bone loss. And for the past 40 or so years, the people of the United States have seen an astounding hike in the number of bone fractures, both in the elderly and in younger people. Adding insult to injury: the incidence of breast and prostate cancers, Crohn's disease, heart disease and premature death are rising, too.

The U.S., an industrialized, educated, world-leading country, is lagging behind other nations in preventative health measures. We are getting sicker, dying younger, and in generally poorer health than dozens of other less wealthy nations. Where is this breakdown occurring? Who is responsible for the decline in Americans' health over the past four decades? On the Glen Beck Show, he quoted that the average cost of health care had risen 78% in the past 6 years according to the Potomac Watch. What really is "Health Care?" I believe it is "Self Care."

Certainly, these issues cannot be whittled down to any one factor. Americans' diets, physical activity patterns, choices about how to use their leisure time, and exposure to multiple environmental contaminants all contribute to the downward spiral. So, too, does a health care system that emphasizes end-stage disease care at enormous fiscal and personal cost, rather than sensible preventive measures.

Still, this book will focus on calcium, the most abundant mineral in the body, as well as the other 17 or so nutrients critical to its absorption. This mineral is an important factor in the big picture of declining health in the U.S. The research I have uncovered and synthesized has linked calcium deficiency to a host of diseases that are plaguing our nation today, leading both old and young people to early suffering, devastating disease and a shortened life span. It has also linked an *overabundance* of the *wrong kind of calcium,* delivered in various forms of supplements and foods, with health issues. In other words: many of us are getting plenty of mostly useless calcium, delivered in forms that don't properly nourish our bones.

So much of what health experts and government agencies advise us to do for optimum dietary health is not, as it turns out, necessarily the best things for our bodies—in fact, some of the dietary guidelines that have been set for us are downright *detrimental.* This is turning out to be true for calcium recommendations. The time is ripe to change course away from reliance on dairy products and mega-supplementation of calcium derived from rocks, chalk and oyster shells. To what?

That's what this book is about.

While I recognize that I am going against the grain in terms of "expert" advice, you will see that abundant research contradicts the guidelines that have been set for our nation. This information somehow doesn't get the attention it deserves. Is it a lack of funding to make this information public? Most definitely. Or is it swept under the rug by strong, well-funded agencies and companies that would have a lot to lose if this information were set free in a media storm?

Ditto: that's what this book is about.

Nutrition research is such a conflicted mess that some experts have advised the public to simply ignore its conclusions and use common sense to figure out what to eat. On any given day, you can find a news piece that tells you exactly the opposite of what's been said yesterday—a conclusion that seems to debunk the one made the day before, which itself seemed to be debunked or debunk numerous other conclusions.

For example, in 2006, vitamin E made a lot of national headlines. One day, reports dictated that vitamin E is an essential vitamin for long-term health. Yet, the very next day, that same statement was retracted, and we were warned to ease up on vitamin E consumption because it might increase our risk of heart problems.

Science labors on towards consensus based on the results of these conflicting studies. From time to time, there are leaks to the public that get turned into recommendations, and medicine and consumers jump on them like lifeboats . . . only to find later on that these recommendations, which seemed to be based on solid science, were basically spurious and possibly harmful.

What—or who—is behind the ever-changing nutrition advice we receive? With vitamins, it is big drug manufacturers and government-run agencies. I'm not suggesting that these organizations are purposely tossing wrenches into nutritional research—just that their attentions and financial backing go towards pharmaceutical research instead, which leaves nutritional research in an underfunded state that makes quality, consistent research difficult to perform. At the same time, agribusiness and processed food manufacturers collaborate with government to push the foods that are most profitable by financing research that makes these foods look far healthier than they would in a less biased research setting. (Can you say, "Got milk?" Or "Tums for calcium?") So: not only is the good research under funded, but the bad research is *over* funded.

So many people are confidently swallowing horse pills of calcium and guzzling low-fat milk, feeling confident that they are protecting their skeletons. They think they are protecting their kids' bones by making sure they eat plenty of dairy foods. They need to change what they are doing—and *right now* is not a moment too soon!

Should we forget about vitamin and mineral pills and try to meet our needs with the foods we eat? Of course, this is our ultimate goal. But there are a few problems with this approach, most importantly that modern agribusiness is reducing drastically the biodiversity and nutrient density of the foods available to us. Even those of us who eat our five to seven vegetable and fruit servings each day and avoid processed grains in favor of whole grains are getting less nutrients per meal than our ancestors did on similar fare.

Used appropriately, appropriate nutritional supplements can benefit us enormously. We don't need to throw out the whole practice of nutrient supplementation because of conflicting studies. We need to dig for correct answers, discovering which studies are impartial and appropriately designed and which are being crafted by the food or vitamin industry to try to pull the wool over our eyes and drive us into buying products that don't really help. We need a reality-based approach that will enable us to make the best possible choices in a world clogged with conflicting evidence.

What perplexes and even angers me is that these conflicting reports and ever-changing directives that are supposedly in our best interest, have led our nation into a state of flux . . . and we stand on the precipice of major health catastrophes. As you continue through this book, you will find out which health conditions are related to intake of calcium—either inadequate intake of the right kind of calcium or intake of *too much* of the *wrong* kind of calcium.

I spent several decades being plagued by chronic illness, beginning with an extremely bad reaction to vaccination in my childhood. After being told that I had a rare blood disease and giving it to my son, I have spent most of my life fighting to find answers to continue to extend our lives. The details are too harrowing and complex to cover in depth here; suffice it to say that mainstream medicine didn't know what to make of us. Many alternative therapies, including magnet therapy (detailed in my book, *Magnetic Miracles*), "real, whole food" nutrition and supplementation, light and sound therapies, strength training and many other were the path that worked the best to bring us to better health. I never gave up-ever!

Being a person who has suffered and been near death with health problems that no Western mainstream doctor could adequately explain or cure, and watching my beloved son suffer too, I felt drawn to utilize and propound alternative therapies in my work. Even though I graduated from college, it was later that I became a staunch researcher and nutritional consultant, and earned a degree in applied magnetic therapy. I am an avid, consumer advocate who wants the truth about our health care system to come out. We can do better and I believe that "Health Care is Self Care." When we have the truth and take action, I believe there is not many health challenges we can't beat. I have seen it numerous times in my own life and in so many others I have worked with.

I remember when my friend Darbe, told me of when her family went to pick up their ailing mother, they could actually feel her bones break! You can imagine how disturbing and scary that must have been for them. And then there was Noba, who had numerous strokes and heart attacks. She would sneeze and break a rib or step down only to fracture another bone in her foot. Poor, precious Ed McMahon the well known sidekick to the late talk show host, Johnny Carson. Little did Ed know that he would live out his last years struggling to hold his head up and constantly have a brace to support his head. The comedian, Phyllis Diller, simply turned her head and broke her neck. This is not funny folks. This is a human tragedy that I have seen over and over in disturbing numbers. With approximately 50,000 women a year dying from fractures related to osteoporosis, and men on track to have more often deadly hip fractures than even women in the next 40 year's or so, a 33% increase in forearm fractures in young kids and up to 50% or so increase in overall fractures in young girls and boys, we should be scared—very scared. And of course, I'll never forget the story I read about in my research about an accomplished dancer who died young, in her early 50's. She used to measure approximately 5'4" tall and when she died she was 4'11" and had died a very, long & painful death. Then there are those who suffer a simple mineral deficiency that causes heart arrhythmia's and potentially die from it because they were never told of such a simple solution. Please let these words wake us up—it's really real!!!! These are *our* sisters, mothers, fathers, brothers, kids, grandparents—they are human beings who deserve the truth and deserve to live their lives in health if they choose to adopt the correct lifestyle and habits.

I found my way to working alongside Norman Cousins, M.D., author of *Anatomy of an Illness* and *Laughter is the Best Medicine* and groundbreaking expert on the link between thoughts and physical health. He was an amazing mentor to me as we collaborated at the Norris Cancer Center, where we worked together and we used simple techniques, like extreme directional breathing, to raise frigid body temperatures in cancer patients and to otherwise cultivate their mind-body connectivity.

When I would see patients' calcium levels rise, I would know they were probably not going to make it. This is well-understood in modern medicine; end-stage cancer often leads to high calcium levels (hypercalcemia) as tumors eat away at bone and release excess calcium into the circulation. Ten to 20 percent of cancer patients and up to 40 percent of those with advanced cancer have hypercalcemia at some point. Excessive fatigue, changes in heart rate, confusion, muscle weakness, loss of appetite, stomach pain, nausea, vomiting, constipation, frequent urination, and dry mouth can all indicate hypercalcemia in a cancer patient. This imbalance of calcium can be deadly if allowed to progress too far.

This phenomenon led me to wonder about the role of calcium in chronic disease and health. I already knew that:

- It's *more than just* calcium that builds bones and is responsible for the approximately 350 metabolic processes in our body's
- Some respected experts, including researchers Colin Campbell of Cornell University and William McDougall MD, were providing excellent evidence to oppose the push to increase dairy and calcium consumption in the U.S. as preventives against osteoporosis.
- Other researchers had found connections between dairy products, by far Americans' most relied-upon source of calcium, and mysterious and ever more common diseases like Crohn's disease and fibromyalgia.
- Links had been drawn between very high calcium intake from processed food and synthetic supplements to certain cancers (most notably, breast and prostate) as well as of higher rates of instant heart attacks in aging women.
- Some issues had been discovered regarding proper absorp-

tion and assimilation in the body of standard-issue calcium supplements.

I decided to delve and ask some tough questions about calcium. This book holds the treasures I found on my search.

Any evidence that calcium supplements or dairy products cause cancer is controversial and—at this point—not conclusive. Still, there are many reasons it may not be in your best interest to rely on dairy for strengthening your bones. There is strong evidence that *more* calcium is not the answer to many of our big health concerns, but that the real solution is *better* calcium. My aim here is to save you money and effort thrown towards the wrong calcium sources, and most importantly to give you the information you need to properly nourish your bones with real sources of calcium and the 17 vitamins and minerals needed to build strong, healthy bones and prevent the devastating diseases related to lack of and poor assimilation, utilization and retention of poor calcium sources. . We *can* get calcium from sources that are more natural to the body and better assimilated.

Because I've learned so much and because even well-intentioned "experts" are misguiding consumers, I felt it was my responsibility to contribute my voice to try to help quash what Harvard University Medical School's newsletter recently called a "silent epidemic"—an epidemic that is threatening our bones, our bodies and the quality of our lives.

In this book we will cover where we are going wrong in not feeding our bones with the absorbable calcium and other essential mineral co-factors, and how changing this course will empower a turnaround in health crises. Yes, there is good news here: it's *not too late* to turn things around, and it's much easier once you are armed with the right information.

The information in this book is so compelling that it will make it easy for you to commit to a plan that will naturally and completely nourish the bone matrix. You will learn about:

- Getting the right amount of calcium and 17 other known needed nutrients (including vitamin D, magnesium, phosphorus, silica, real vitamin C, selenium, and lysine, . . .) rich in co-factors from wonderful whole foods
- Identifying symptoms of deficiencies and utilizing the list of foods rich in the needed nutrients with the Food & Symptom Chart
- Creating your ideal 15 Minute Whole Body Bone-Building Exercise Program—one that focuses on strengthening and helping to heal your most vulnerable areas
- Avoiding "calcium robbers"—foods and drugs that drain precious calcium and other bone-building minerals from your body
- Using Fast, Easy Recipes rich in the foods abundant with the nutrients needed to build strong bones as well as assist in the 350 or so metabolic processes calcium is needed for
- Knowing who you can count on as allies in the food industry—and those from whom you can expect lies, manipulations, and deceit

This book will give you the tools you need to understand and live what I call a *Whole Body Bone Building lifestyle*. The devastating future of fragile, broken bones and life-shortening diseases can be thwarted. Turn the page and begin today. It's never too soon, and it's never too late.

Wishing you abundant health, happiness & blessings always,

—Catie J. Norris

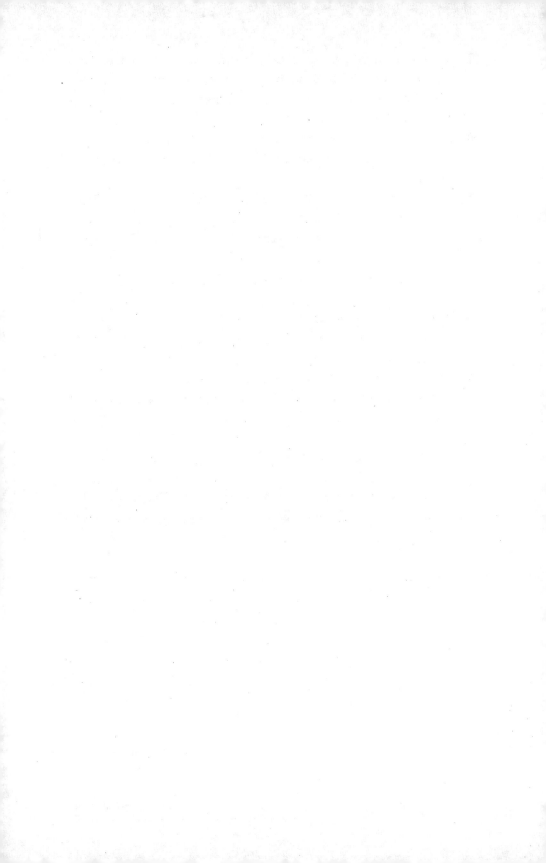

Chapter One

Eat a Rock Lately?

THE TRUTH ABOUT CALCIUM SUPPLEMENTS

You want strong bones that will last a lifetime. That's easy—right? Just take those giant calcium horse pills. As long as you get your 1,200 to 1,500 or more milligrams of calcium a day from those chalky white pills, you'll be doing all you can to prevent osteoporosis. Right?

Sounds easy, but there are definite problems with this approach. Let's try an analogy to explain at least a small part of these problems. If you want your car to go, you have to put gas in it. Where do you put the gas? Do you take a big bucket of petroleum, pop your car's hood, and pour the smelly stuff all over the engine, hoping it'll end up where it needs to go? Of course you don't. You put the gas in the gas tank, exactly where it needs to be to do its job.

As it turns out, swallowing a big horse pill of non-absorbable calcium is more like the first approach than the latter. Instead of putting it in the bones, where you want it, you're pouring it into the body, where it seems to accumulate in the bloodstream, at least temporarily. This may not turn out to be a good thing. Just as pouring gasoline onto an engine just might create untoward ill effects (bad smells, smoke, and a car that doesn't run because the gas tank is still empty), pouring loads of calcium into your body seems to create some problems.

One study published in the *British Medical Journal* in early 2008 highlights one such possible problem. In New Zealand, researchers gathered 1,471 healthy postmenopausal women, 55 and over. They wanted to test a hypothesis that calcium supplements would help prevent heart attacks, strokes, and sudden death from cardiovascular (heart) disease. Past studies had found that calcium supplements positively affected cholesterol counts; other research suggests very small blood pressure-lowering and weight loss effects—all changes that could protect the heart. It seemed like a slam-dunk that there would be some benefit of calcium supplements on the heart.

The women got either calcium supplements (a total of 1000 mg of calcium citrate) or placebo pills daily for about five years, and their calcium intake from food was also measured. Imagine the horror of these researchers when they computed their data and found that the group of women who took calcium pills had *higher* incidence of heart attacks, strokes, and sudden death compared to the women taking the placebo! It wasn't a hugely increased incidence—but it was significant.

The calcium did have mild benefit in terms of protecting bone, but the risk of heart problems or stroke seemed to outweigh that benefit. In the five years of this study, prevention of one symptomatic bone fracture required treating 50 women with calcium. To cause a heart attack, the investigators concluded, they needed only to treat 44 women with calcium; and to cause a stroke required treating 56 women with calcium. Not great risk-to-benefit odds. Even one precious life is too much.

The bulk of research studies on calcium supplements (carbonates, citrates, phosphates, gluconates, coral calcium, . . .) demonstrates that such supplements don't seem to protect the bones against osteoporosis or related conditions nearly as well as we might expect, based on the calcium recommendations given to us by the medical establishment. And if calcium supplements turn out to have significant *risks,* too, as suggested by the *British Medical Journal* study described above, we could be facing some big problems.

One of our country's top (former) Cardiologists, Gary Gordon, M.D., of the Gordon Research Institute in Scottsdale, AZ shared a story that has given me shivers and unending nightmares. He spoke of his experience over the years, when doing open heart surgery; he would see this disturbing build up in and around his patient's heart and vascular system that he had to *cut through and peel off* with a pliers like surgical tool. Could it be that the calcium mineral salt supplements (*hard, inert minerals*) that these precious people consumed, the fortified foods, as well as other lifestyle choices, may have been fossilizing him or her? Read on to find your answers.

As we continue to eat convenient, "enriched" boxed foods, altered foods, fast foods, and synthetic nutrients, we are the 2nd, 3rd, and 4th generations suffering from this serious adulterated life style and foods. Many Doctors are quoted in Mary Frost, M.A.'s book "Going Back to the Basics of Human Health" stating that in fact, the synthetic nutrient manufacturer's and distributor's have not told of their often poisonous effects.

This is not to say that you should jettison the whole idea of taking a calcium supplement. If you are taking a calcium supplement to fortify your bones and prevent bone loss, you're on the right track; but if you are taking in the wrong kind of hard-to-absorb calcium, you may actually be absorbing only a fraction of the calcium you take in, or you may be putting too much calcium into your bloodstream that can't be utilized by the body. To revisit our car metaphor, you not only have to get the gasoline from the pump into the gas tank; you also have to use the right kind of gasoline.

Calcium is not really bad for your heart, but the *kind* of calcium you take into your body matters to the health of your cardiovascular system. As it turns out, calcium absorption is a tricky business, and it can make or break (literally!) the health of your bones. Even if you religiously pop your calcium pills every day, despite your good intentions, your bones just might be getting *totally ripped off* because it most likely is a poorly synthesized calcium mineral salt that has been chemically maneuvered to create a chemical reaction—much like a drug does in the body.

Bone Health and Calcium 101

Taking a supplement takes a lot less thinking and energy than planning for a well-balanced diet day after day. But no supplement can protect against the ill effects of a diet that fails to nourish our bodies or fulfill its most fundamental needs. Americans are now paying the price for poor dietary choices with higher incidences of a long laundry list of chronic diseases. In particular, poor mineral nutrition—the subject of this book—is linked with:

Acne	Agoraphobia, Panic & Anxiety
Arrythmias	Bone Fractures
Bone Pain	Colon & Rectal Cancers
Cramps	Craving Salt & Carbohydrates—
Crohn's Disease	yet intolerant to them, ...
Early Death	Decayed Teeth
Hormone Imbalances	High Blood Pressure
Irregular Nerve Impulses	Hypertension
Metabolic Weight Gain	Joint Pain
Mottled, Brown Teeth	Mitro Valve Prolapse
Osteoporosis	Muscle Pain (local & systemic)
Poor Connective Tissue	Poor Blood Clotting
Poor Moods	Poor Insulin Production
Rickets	Poor Sleep (Insomnia)
Thin Jaws & Wrists	Strokes
Twitching	Tingling/Numbing

Most hip fractures are due to osteoporosis, a disease where bone is unable to mineralize and deteriorates, becoming increasingly weak and porous. Osteoporosis is caused by many factors, including hormonal changes following menopause (in women), lack of weight-bearing exercise, and poor diet.

The most dreaded and deadly consequence of weak, porous bones is hip fracture. If you are female and white, your chance of a hip fracture in your lifetime is two to three times that of a man's. Your overall lifetime chance of hip fracture: one in seven, with a doubling of your risk each five to six years after your 50th birthday.

Almost *one in four women* who fracture a hip die from complications in the ensuing months. The cost of treating a hip fracture averages just under $27,000, and the American Academy of Orthopedic Surgeons predicts that by the year 2050, Americans will suffer 650,000 hip fractures a year—*that's almost 1,800 a day!* Over 25 percent of people who experience a hip fracture will become immobilized as a result. That's 450 people *a day*, relegated to life in wheelchairs and beds by osteoporosis.

This health crisis is not limited to the elderly or to women, either. The ages are getting younger and younger: a woman has a 50 percent chance of a bone fracture after the age of 50 years. Current research shows that the incidence of male hip fractures is rising steeply. As a matter of fact, men will have higher rates of hip fractures in the next 20 to 30 years than even women.

Although the medical mainstream has put forth the impression that preventing osteoporosis is as simple as guaranteeing calcium adequacy and getting some weight-bearing exercise, a great deal is still not known. It and the government continue to send out authoritative edicts about calcium and dairy consumption: daily calcium requirements, two glasses of milk a day.

But the far less cut-and-dried truth is that there is huge controversy about the roles of calcium and our most common dietary source of calcium, dairy products, in osteoporosis prevention. Intake of calcium, most certainly, does not tell the whole story.

THE BONE REMODELING PROCESS AND THE ROLE OF CALCIUM

From before birth, even as our bodies formed in our mothers' wombs, our bodies have built and broken down bone cells. A growing child, obviously, is building more bone than is being broken down. In our young adult years, bone building continues; in middle age, the rate of bone renewal more or less matches the rate of breakdown. As levels of bone-building hormones drop in late middle age, loss of bone begins to surpass building of new bone. If you've been doing everything right, your bones reached a high maximum density while you were young, and you have enough to spare that you'll never suffer a broken bone from osteoporosis. Fewer and fewer Americans fit this mold, however.

This process of bone building and breakdown is also known as the *bone remodeling cycle*. Bone *resorption* describes the natural breakdown and removal of bone tissue, and bone *formation* is another term used for bone building. Specialized cells called *osteoclasts* on the surface of bone dissolve bone cells, creating small holes, which *osteoblasts*—another kind of cell—then fill with new bone. When in balance, this process maintains strong, healthy bone. When bone remodeling falls out of balance in favor of bone resorption—the usual situation for Americans—*osteopenia*, or pre-osteoporosis, and the final insult of osteoporosis are the end results.

A diagnosis of osteopenia is a last chance to avoid osteoporosis. It refers to decreased bone mineral density as seen on a bone scan, and often elicits a sigh of relief: *oh, great, at least it's not osteoporosis!* But significant bone has already been lost by this point. It's time to get on the Whole Body Bone-Building Bandwagon, and quick.

Although getting enough calcium in the right forms is important for bone health, *there is a good deal more to the bone remodeling equation than calcium adequacy.* To properly assimilate and utilize calcium, your body needs a whole spectrum of other (17 or so according to research) minerals such as magnesium to help calcium be absorbed properly, manganese-crucial to make a strong bone, boron helps keep calcium in the body, and others may make up the protein matrix in the bone, while others are important to support that process. It's not just calcium! It needs vitamin D. It needs weight-bearing exercise and it needs to be free of bone-robbing influences that tip the balance towards resorption.

Keep in mind that your alkali reserves originate in your bones. Your bones should be be rich in the minerals and nutrients needed for strong bones, and the many other life giving processes. Whatever your age, if you do not get enough daily replenishment of premium calcium, as well as the needed minerals and cofactors, your body automatically pulls calcium out of your "bone bank" to cover urgent needs elsewhere in the body. Silently, the calcium robbing crisis takes place within the skeletal structure, producing no warning signs until bones begin snapping like twigs. This usually does not happen until after middle age (only in this day and age, but this did not occur 100 years ago). Unfortunately, certain pharmaceutical drugs meant to strengthen bones, are now being cited for "spontaneous femur fractures" just from standing on their legs!

Bone loss is happening to younger and younger people as diets deliver less and less bioavailable, usable mineral nutrition and as we spend more time sitting. Those who do not exercise and who consume a lot of "bone-robber" foods or medications may have too slow a rate of bone building in youth, setting them up to have less to lose in old age. A teenaged girl who drinks 32-ounces of dark sodas every day and gets little to no exercise is robbing herself of prime bone-building time, and her risk of osteoporosis later in life is higher. (See Tufts University Study regarding dark sodas and bone loss). She may have very serious consequences that can effect her and her potential offspring also.

Dr. David A. Steenblock, D.O. of Personalized Regenerative Medicine in Mission Viejo, CA says that a proper bone building lifestyle and wholesome nourishment is crucial early in life and throughout as strong bone mineralization is vital to build stem cells in the bone marrow. Stem cells are contained in your body and used to help heal ones aches & pains. As we age and suffer from health challenges such as osteoarthritis, heart attacks, multiple sclerosis, ... our stem cells are needed and can even be extracted from the bones and injected into the blood stream to help dramatically heal these diseases.

What shifts in middle age to so strongly affect bone remodeling? As mentioned earlier, the shift is partially hormonal, especially for women. Renowned Osteoporosis researcher, Professor Heaney from Creighton University, in Omaha, NE, told me that research has shown that the influence is less than we have been led to believe and that it could average around 15% for most women throughout menopause. The hormones estrogen and progesterone are instrumental bone-builders. As levels of those hormones drop, so does the rate of bone-building in a woman's body. This rapid loss of hormonal stimulation of bone-building is the reason why women develop osteoporosis more than men do.

Hormones tell part of the story, but not all of it. A woman can strengthen her bones, starting young, enough to protect herself after menopause. Good nutrition, including quality, bioavailable calcium sources, is every bit as important as hormone balance; so is a workout program you can stick with day-to-day for the rest of your days.

It is vital to learn all you can about supplemental calcium sources so that you don't suffer the consequences of taking useless, inadequate supplements. With the right information, you won't throw your money away on supplements that are only minimally absorbable. You won't be led down the garden path to believing that your bones are getting all the calcium and mineral cohorts needed to prevent and combat bone loss from poorly absorbed calcium.

The going popular belief about osteoporosis is that it is caused by lack of calcium in the diet, and that if we guzzle enough low-fat milk or swallow enough calcium pills, we can protect ourselves. In these pages, you'll learn that the picture of osteoporosis and related conditions isn't quite so simple. Although calcium is crucial for strong bones—the right kind of calcium, in the right amounts from the right sources—there are many other factors to attend to in a comprehensive bone-protective program. And the sources of calcium commonly used in an attempt to nourish bones tend to fall short.

Figure 1.1: Healthy vs. Malnourished Bone

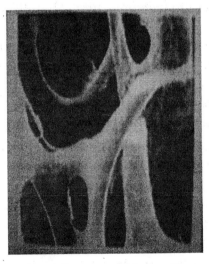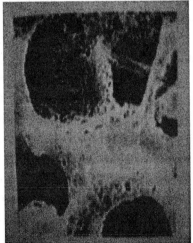

Healthy bone is on the left; malnourished, acidified bone is to the right.

STRONGER BONES . . . WITH DRUGS? NO THANKS!

The quick-fix answer for the osteopenia and osteoporosis epidemic in the U.S.? Drugs, of course! As the incidence of osteoporosis soars, drugs designed to preserve bone mass in women at risk are becoming increasingly big sellers in the pharmaceutical market. Several classes of drugs have been developed to try to counter this devastating disease.

The most-prescribed of these are the *bisphosphonates,* which are designed to slow resorption. This drug class includes Fosamax, Boniva, Actonel, and Reclast. Related drugs that are not bisphosphonates but that work to slow resorption include Fortical, Micalcin, Nolvadex, and Evista. A few drugs both slow resorption and increase bone building: hormone replacement therapy including estrogen, sold as Premarin or estradiol, and parathyroid hormone, sold as a drug called Forteo.

These drugs do help some people initially. The bisphosphonates reduce risk of hip and spine fractures by about 50 percent. At this writing, Evista has been shown to increase bone density in short-term studies, but its longer-term ability to prevent fractures hasn't yet been proven. Hormone replacement with drugs like Premarin also help build and preserve bone. But all of these work at a cost. There are always risks to consider.

Bisphosphonates' more common side effects include nausea, abdominal pain, or irritation or erosion of the inner lining of the esophagus. These drugs also triple the risk of a rare problem called *bone necrosis,* where blood supply is cut off to sections of bone, leading to death of bone tissue and permanent disability. Evista brings increased risk of blood clots, as well as risk of abdominal pain, arthritis, depression, diarrhea, fever, gas, gynecological problems, urinary tract infections, sinusitis, sore throat, headache, hot flashes, cough, weight gain, indigestion, nausea, and other stomach and intestinal problems. Nolvadex—which is actually tamoxifen, the estrogen-blocking breast cancer drug—can cause hot flashes, stomach upset, vaginal discharge or dryness, and hypercalcemia (!), and increases the risk of uterine cancer, endometriosis (where the uterine lining that is shed each month during the menstrual period spreads outside of the uterus, causing pain and heavy periods), and uterine fibroids (benign tumors). And standard hormone replacement therapy with Premarin (a form of estrogen made from the urine of pregnant mares) and progestin (a drug that resembles the female hormone progesterone) has been found unsafe for long-term use due to increases in risk of breast cancer—which makes it unsafe for use as an osteoporosis preventative, a use for which it was touted for many years. Can you imagine the number of casualties this may have had?! Whose dear friend was a victim, whose sister, whose mother? Are we so numb that we lack the compassion that is needed to stir our emotions to possible change or maybe we don't have the time or think we can't make a difference?!

When it seems like it is too late, riddled with deteriorating bones, we often find ourselves in a corner, believing that we need to do the drugs. You *do* have a choice and *it is yours* and yours only. Our fear often keeps us immobilized and keeps us from making the appropriate choice for our true bone building. We need to take a deep breath and deepen our faith. (Sometimes—to do nothing is doing something until you have had a chance to digest the whole picture.) We need to develop this *faith* to give us *hope* so that we can develop the wisdom to find our best choices and take action! Action?! We're so used to being told what should be best for us and after years of disappointments, you'd think we'd stop going to the same source for the "right" answers. If we can't make a plan *together* with our health care provider, than it may be a great opportunity to explore other allies. I am amazed at what people have fallen for but even more amazed at the fact that these drugs can be marketed to innocent souls looking for answers and that the drug companies are able to promote something with such devastating side effects and often times with very low success rate. Unfortunately, most of us don't have a plan for our health so we fit into someone else's plan that may not be the best for us. We're often too lazy (I was there at one time!) to take the action we need because it was "so easy" taking someone else's advice and taking that pill they advised!

If the bone deterioration is so far advanced, it is doubtful that the risks of drugs may be adequately counteracted by benefits. Utilizing synthetic sources to bring life to our bones and body hasn't shown the results that they should have and sooner or later we will all have to admit this. This is a crucial time and our decisions will determine our quality of life and often times our length of life. The building blocks of our bodies have always been real, live, whole foods—they are natural sources, that are most *absorbed*, best *utilized* in the body and that can be retained in the bones with the appropriate supporting minerals. Why would we think that we could duplicate Mother Nature? When I have found my back to the wall, fighting for my life, I have found many of my most profound answers in my kitchen & garden. I utilized the most potent, most nutritious live foods & whole food supplements, super foods and herbs rich in the *real nutrients* proven to help cleanse, strengthen, nourish, nurture, and help heal my cells that just happen to make up my tissue, glands, organs, veins, arteries, muscles, and *bones!* My prayers are that you never find yourself in this place. Hopefully, you are still in a place where you can make a huge difference simply by living a whole body bone building lifestyle—a lifestyle that includes the use of a "real" food calcium supplement. Keep in mind that it is never too late no matter where you are.

SUPPLEMENTS: A "NATURAL" ALTERNATIVE TO MEDICATIONS?

Nutritional supplements are widely considered to be natural medicines. The vitamins and minerals sold in most stores are advertised as being identical to those found in healthy foods. But what are those pills packed with calcium, vitamin C, B vitamins, and the like really made out of? Where do those nutrients actually come from?

As it turns out, in most supplements, these supplements are composed of crushed rocks processed with industrial chemicals; petroleum derivatives; oils; hydrogenated acetone-processed sugars; and/or irradiated animal fats.

This may sound unbelievable to you, but it's true. Despite label claims that a supplement is natural, the ingredients inside are almost always synthetic. They are *created*, not derived from natural sources like nutrient-dense foods.

CALCIUM 101

Calcium is the most abundant mineral in the body. Ninety-nine percent of the calcium in the body is found in the bones, bound up with phosphorus in the form of *hydroxyapatite* crystals. This is the body's storage depot for calcium. The other one percent plays a number of important roles in the bloodstream and soft tissues, including:

- Cofactor for proteins and enzymes. This means that calcium naturally bonds with proteins and enzymes to help them take the vitamins and minerals where they need to go.
- Blood pressure. Here, calcium plays a pivotal role in the constriction and relaxation of blood vessels.
- Hormone production. Calcium affects secretion of insulin and other hormones. (The pancreas can't make insulin without calcium)
- The action of muscles. Muscle cannot contract or relax without calcium.

Once it enters the body, calcium is supposed to travel into the small intestine, where it is then absorbed into the bloodstream. When poorly absorbed sources are used, a lot of the calcium taken in may pass right through the body in the digestive tract, going out in fecal matter without ever being absorbed or worse yet, it may find its way throughout the body getting stuck in the wrong places as the latest study's are now showing.

Whatever calcium your body has managed to absorb through the intestinal wall into the bloodstream is circulated throughout the body so that it can be taken up at the cellular level. Whatever calcium is not used by bone, muscle, or other tissues is filtered out by the kidneys and excreted in urine.

Calcium exists in nature only in combination with other substances or "compounds." In supplement form, several different calcium compounds are used, including calcium carbonate, calcium phosphate, calcium gluconate, calcium citrate, and coral calcium to name a few of the most popular. The actual amount of calcium in the supplement depends on the different amounts of elemental calcium found in the compound.

I know how hard it is to interpret the compound derivatives found on the labels of the different kinds of calcium supplements. Even for someone who understands nutrition pretty darned well, choosing the right calcium can be downright *confusing*. When I set out to choose the best possible calcium supplement for my family, I learned how much I *didn't* know. While I carefully read labels, I didn't really know what the ingredients were. I didn't understand the various kinds of calcium. Should I purchase calcium carbonate or calcium citrate? What source is the calcium derived from—pure or synthetic? How much is needed to meet the daily recommended amounts for the various ages and genders in my family? How much calcium is actually available to be absorbed by my body? Is it best to take calcium all at once or spread throughout the day? I had so many questions—and very few answers.

It soon became my mission to decipher the ingredients list so I could make an informed and wise choice from the dazzling selection of calcium supplements. I think I've been fairly successful in figuring it all out, and share this knowledge with you in these pages. In Chapter Five, I outline whole foods that are rich in easily-absorbed calcium and all the minerals that are crucial to the approximately 350 different metabolic processes these nutrients contribute to in the body, as well as what to look for in a calcium supplement to feed your bones, not rob them of calcium and other essential minerals.

There's another reason your choice of calcium is important. When your bones, intestines and the kidney are unable to process calcium, dangerous levels of calcium begin to *linger* in the bloodstream rather than entering the bones where it is needed most. This increase in blood calcium levels is called hypercalcemia, which is thought to be associated with some serious diseases. This could partially explain the increase in cardiovascular deaths in the calcium study mentioned at the opening of this chapter. We'll return to this topic later on.

What's in YOUR Calcium Supplement?

While we are educated and directed to take calcium supplements, the majority of those available to us aren't providing our bones with any benefits. In fact, many of these supplements are flooding our blood streams, creating unhealthy levels of serum calcium.

Common forms of calcium found in most over-the-counter calcium supplements are composed of elements that are easily absorbed by plants, but not by people. As you continue to read, you will discover why these over the counter sources are setting us up for major health catastrophes.

Like so many things in our world, this stark contrast comes down to cost factors. Supplement manufacturers derive calcium from free resources and mass-produce it in ways that are cost-effective and profit-building. The problem is that consumers are not getting the absorbable, beneficial dose of calcium needed for bones to support them over a lifetime. Let's examine

---

GET THE LEAD OUT . . . OF OUR CALCIUM SUPPLEMENTS!

(From http://www.nrdc.org/nrdc/status/hecalsr.html)

In January 1997, the Natural Resources Defense Council took action under California's law, and reached an agreement under which Leiner Health Products Group, the nation's largest manufacturer of dietary calcium supplements, will manufacture virtually lead-free calcium products. Leiner uses a process called chelation to remove lead—a feat that other manufacturers have claimed isn't feasible.

Environmentalists and health advocates hoped that the Leiner settlement would set a precedent, and force other manufacturers to "get the lead out." Unfortunately, in April 1997 the California Attorney General compromised the public's health and reached a settlement with several manufacturers allowing them to sell calcium products for the next two years, without warning labels, with exposures of up to 6 micrograms for supplements and up to 9 micrograms for antacids. The settlement did propose lead reductions after two years, *but even after that time*, these manufacturers were able to avoid compliance if they could show that it would cause an increase in prices. This is a sad proposal for the masses of unsuspecting consumers who have no idea if they are or have been consuming supplements laden with lead. Please note that Leiner products are mass marketed to many large chain stores nationwide.

---

the calcium choices found in most supplement products—some of which I'm willing to bet are in *your* medicine cabinet.

The most popular forms of calcium are *calcium citrate* (derived from oyster shell), *calcium carbonate* (derived from chalk and rock) and *microcrystalline hydroxyapatite* (derived from cow bone). Every one of these forms of calcium can be billed as 100 percent natural.

Stop and think about this for a moment. What's natural about taking a shell, bone, chalk, rock or industrialized chemical and then putting it into a big machine to be pulverized into a powder or tablet? And this is not where the process stops. Those big, "natural" calcium pills you swallow are processed further—*much* further.

Some might say it's time to examine the way we use the word "natural" when we talk about food and nutritional supplements. A spoon full of highly refined white sugar? 100 percent natural! High-fructose corn syrup? Also natural—just because it happens to be derived from plants. Ingenious marketing, but we're talking about some of the most highly processed stuff imaginable. Most calcium supplements—most supplements in general—are equally processed and equally unnatural.

Still not convinced? Let's take a look at a few of these so-called "natural" calcium supplements: where they come from and how they are produced.

Calcium Citrate

This form has been touted as one of the better absorbed sources today. Here's how calcium citrate supplements are made: citric acid is usually derived by adding cultures of a mold, *Aspergillus niger,* to a medium containing rocks or oyster shells and sugar in the form of either sucrose (table sugar) or glucose (the simplest form of sugar). The sugar usually comes from corn or molasses. The mold digests the sugars to make citric acid, and is then filtered out; the resulting substance is then precipitated with lime to make calcium citrate salt. This salt is then turned back into citric acid by treating it with sulfuric acid.

When blended, the calcium carbonate and citric acid create free calcium and free carbonate. The citric acid also breaks in half, creating free citrate and free acid. Now, in this soup of chemicals, you have four separated components that have to regroup. Doesn't exactly make you think of natural sources and processes, does it?

The acid and the carbon bond together to form carbon dioxide, which is a gas. Then the mixture starts bubbling out carbon dioxide, leaving only two remaining components: calcium and citrate. Forced to bond, they form what is known as calcium citrate. But remember, this newly formed calcium started out as rocks, chalk or oyster shells and citric acid.

And this is what is sold as a "natural" source for calcium. No big surprise that calcium citrate is only about 30 to 35 percent absorbed in the human gastrointestinal tract.

Calcium Carbonate

Calcium carbonate is a quite popular form of this mineral found in supplements. It's made from limestone or chalk, and is used in the manufacture of paint, rubber, plastic, ceramics, putty, polishes, insecticides, and inks; it's also used as a filler for adhesives, matches, pencils, crayons, linoleum, insulating compounds, and welding rods. Amazing-huh?!

Calcium carbonate's absorption rate can be as low as 22 percent (Patrick, 1999). Although the least expensive form and a best seller, calcium carbonate is now coming under fire by some respected scientists. Dr. Robert P. Heaney, principal scientist at Creighton Osteoporosis Research Center, and Dr. Pierre J. Meunier, a French researcher, believe calcium carbonate may block *most* of the absorption of the mineral phosphorus. This is critical because phosphorous makes up *more than half* the mass of bone mineral!

Dr. Heaney suggests that "the best way to help our patients meet their needs is to use a source that provides both calcium and phosphorous, such as dairy products and/or a calcium-phosphate supplement." (Heaney 2002).

However: before you go running for that gallon of skim milk in your fridge, you should know that dairy products may not be a good bet for bone health. More on this in Chapter 3. Also, keep in mind that neither calcium citrate nor calcium carbonate can be absorbed without a number of other nutrients, including vitamin D and specific pH factors. Keep in mind that we can absorb many things that may not be good for us like poison. It's more than absorption as you will see soon.

If you were to look at the labels on most calcium supplements, I guarantee you will find the majority contain calcium carbonate, calcium citrate or coral calcium listed as the top ingredient. Or it may be a fizzy drink from calcium gluconate. Don't be fooled; this is just a fancy way of saying "mineral salts." Many of the so-called "natural" products on the market contain processed rocks known as mineral salts. These mineral salts are not meant for human consumption, nor are they meeting human nutritional needs. *Mineral salts are not a natural part of the human food chain.*

Calcium Gluconate

This form of calcium is calcium carbonate processed with gluconic acid (a substance used in cleaning compounds). It's used in sewage purification and to keep coffee powders from caking. This is often in a fizzy, fruit flavored drink that is marketed to be better absorbed because of its liquidity and chemical processing. Just one infomercial company has sold over a 100 million dollars of this product with a doctor professing its virtues.

Coral Calcium

How about coral calcium—a form that has been relentlessly hyped in some alternative health circles (this infomercial sold over 200 million dollars in product before being pulled off the T.V.)! To hear the claims made by proponents of this calcium, which is made from the limestone shells of coral reef bits that have fallen off of coral reefs around Okinawa, Japan, it is the reason for Okinawan longevity and the cure for a long list of diseases, including cancer. Truth be told, coral calcium is mostly the same kind of calcium found in over-the-counter antacids and cheap calcium carbonate calcium pills—although it costs far, far more. Independent tests have found lead in coral calcium, as well as in calcium supplements from oyster shell. And all the hype over coral calcium, including a long laundry list of false claims as to its healing power, has gotten several of its proponents into big trouble with the FDA.

Corals themselves are actually tiny animals that are related to jellyfish and sea anemones. Coral forms into a hard skeleton of calcium carbonate that serves as a protective layer. As coral dies, new generations emerge to grow on top of the calcium carbonate remains which in turn form a coral reef. A calcium supplement obtained from coral is actually from crushed rock, also known as . . . mineral salts.

Furthermore, not all of the trace elements found in coral calcium, such as cadmium, uranium, and mercury, are appropriate for the human body. Once this inorganic synthetic calcium-containing material is ingested, the body has to scramble to adapt to this foreign substance, which ultimately taxes the system. Just for the record, recent literature from one of the largest marketers of Coral Calcium has a new story behind their coral wonder: "they also found that when coral sand was used as a fertilizer, crops improved as well." So the plants digested the hard inert coral sand first and than the humans . . . this was an important last step that has been the missing link in most of the supplements on the market. A serious missing link that may have helped changed the healthy history of millions of people. More on that later.

DOSAGE DECEPTION

According to Susan E. Brown, PhD, CNS, our nation tends to ingest 1,000 to 1,500 milligrams of calcium daily to maintain bone health, while other populations that tend to eat a plant-based diet maintain strong bones with a daily calcium intake of 400 mg or less. The World Health Organization recommends 400–500 mg per day. One of the biggest, if not biggest, study's done on diet and how it effects our health was the The China Study (or Project). This was a monumental study from Cornell & Oxford University's which showed a population in rural China who didn't have the serious health challenges that we have in this country due to their diet and lifestyle. This included osteoporosis, heart disease, diabetes, . . . This study showed how these lovely people got 300 to 500 mgs of calcium (and other vital nutrients and mineral) from their food and showed normal, natural bone thinning and much reduced disease process in their body's. This must really surprise you as we have been constantly told we need much more.

Walter Willett, professor at the Harvard School of Public Health and chairman of its nutrition department, says that "there is no evidence that we have a calcium emergency, as the dairy industry would have us believe." Marion Nestle of NYU, chairperson of the nutrition and food studies department there as well as a member of the FDA's science advisory board, put it this way after the government raised daily recommendations for calcium for teens and people over 50 to 1,200 and 1,300 mg per day, respectively: "I think it's amazing to have set the calcium requirements so high."

Do Americans really need three times more calcium than the rest of the world? Of course not. The depletion we face is not in the *amount* of calcium we consume, but in the *forms* we consume.

Calcium supplements can and should play a role in promoting bone health, but the truth is that the vast majority of calcium supplements available to American consumers are woefully inadequate—even risky, because of the effects they have on your body's access to other minerals that are equally important for bone health. Crucial differences in sources for calcium and the appropriate inclusion of complementary mineral bone-builders can deeply impact how well—or poorly—your bones survive your "golden years."

Despite the fact that Americans are consuming more calcium than other nations, we are facing higher rates of osteoporosis and deaths related to falls. Our nutrient-deficient diets, combined with bone-leaching substances such as stress, sunscreen (blocking out the benefits of natural vitamin D), processed foods, alcohol, bone leaching medications, lack of exercise and excess salt have left

Americans' bones running on empty. This has led to many health challenges and diseases related to this poor lifestyle:

Acid Reflux	Acne
Brown Teeth	Colon/Rectal Cancer
Connective Tissue Disorders (ribs popping out)	Decayed Teeth
Diabetes, Hypertension	Fractures
Kidney stones	Mottle Teeth
Heart Arrythmias	Osteomylitis (Thinning jaw)
Osteopenia (precursor to Osteoporosis)	Osteoporosis (poorly mineralized bones)
Receding Gums	Rickets (soft bones)
Strokes	

PLANTS CAN DIGEST ROCKS . . . AND PEOPLE CAN DIGEST PLANTS

So, if dairy isn't the answer, what is? Calcium supplements made from rocks and shells. . . . right?

We know for a fact that plants can *miraculously* dig deep into to the earth and extract these hard, inert minerals and break them down and absorb essential minerals in rock form that enable them to grow and thrive. *Humans cannot.* This is evident when you consider the paradox that plagues the U.S. today. To better understand why people have such trouble absorbing and utilizing chalk, stones, and shells to feed their bones, let's take a close look at the food chain.

Plants make their own food from raw materials in soil, using essential enzymes and soil-based mineral salts. Once natural metabolic processes occur within those plants, the minerals no longer exist as mineral salts; they have been digested by the plant. Various organic sequences take place that alter the mineral salts, using various carbohydrates, lipids and proteins that are present in the plant. Using these minerals, photosynthesis, enzymes and other natural occurrences, plants are able to produce vitamins required for life.

The next step in the food chain is for humans to consume these plants to get their nutrition. This is the key—the missing link: *we are designed to absorb calcium from plants, not from rocks or oyster shells or chemical soups made from these inorganic substances.*

However, that is not what is happening in today's modern world. The food chain seems to have broken precisely at that link, and this

---

STAGGERING INCREASE IN CLEFT PALATE DISEASE

Description of cleft palate—Columbia Encyclopedia

"incomplete fusion of bones of the **palate**. The **cleft** may be confined to the soft **palate** at the back of the mouth; it may include the hard **palate**, or roof of the mouth; or it may extend through the gum and lip, producing a gap in the teeth and a **cleft** lip, which **is** cosmetically difficult to repair but **is** not disabling" It occurs in one of 600 to 800 births and often found in third world country's. There are nutritional deficiency's associated with this malady such as B6 and folate to name a few. A "toxic overload" of Vitamin A (fat soluble form) has been linked to this disfiguring disease also.

It is fortunate for charity programs like Operation Smile that help bring normalcy to many of these children with the help of many dedicated Doctor's, health practitioner's, and volunteers to operate and reform the effected area—all for a nominal fee of approximately $250. (Please see references if you would like to change a child's life forever.)

Because we need calcium and numerous other minerals to build (or "re-build") strong bones, it is critical to provide the body with appropriate nutrition and minerals when preparing for a bone graft so that it can heal optimally.

---

is one reason why we are seeing alarming increases of diseases that are literally killing us in staggering amounts each year.

This is partially due to the simple fact that most people don't eat enough plants. But even those who are genuinely concerned about their health and make an effort to eat enough plants are adversely affected by changes in the production and processing of food over the past two centuries. Not only have we contaminated the soil where plants grow, our Western ways of processing foods, refining whole grains, and immersing food in preservatives to extend the shelf life of products are all contributing to a stripped-down, dramatically reduced intake of essential vitamins, minerals and enzymes.

To combat the effects of our fast-paced, industrialized world, health and longevity seekers have been turning to supplements in an effort to provide their bodies with vitamins, minerals and herbs. In part, this strategy is meant to offset the nutritional deficiencies related to eating an unbalanced diet. This movement away from eating whole foods in their natural state to swallowing a handful of pills is where, I believe, one of the biggest breakdown is occurring.

Although the rationale for snapping up extra nutrients from the supermarket supplement aisle is sound, the truth is that a vast majority of the supplements out there are synthetic. Even if the molecules of the B vitamins in that B vitamin tablet somewhat match those found in healthy whole foods, they are usually bound to other molecules that do not normally accompany them in those foods, and they are missing all of the complementary nutrients that occur in the nutrient's matrix in food form. They are merely attempts to copy nature's nutrients. Unfortunately, they usually come from industrialized chemicals and often contain petroleum which can't be broken down by the body. When a person swallows synthetic supplements, they are continuing this pattern of "breaking the food chain" by moving farther away from nature's whole food strategy. Instead of ingesting chemical elements that are virtually bursting with life, we are allowing synthetic *imposters* into our systems.

CEDAR SINAI HOSPITAL PHYSICIAN'S CASE STUDY:

A 65 year old woman diagnosed with osteoporosis advised to go on pharmaceutical drug to strengthen bones decides to use plant supplement rich in calcium that included numerous other minerals. Clinical indications found increases in several different bone markers but in her most vulnerable hip area the increase was 10.7% alone. Her Doctor called her after the 14 month of monitoring and left the message, "Whatever you are taking, continue with it!"

I've always been an avid naturalist and supplement enthusiast. I still am! But, I've found that what we *choose* to ingest is as important as shaking the pill out of the bottle and swallowing it—it's actually *more* important.

HYPERCALCEMIA: DANGEROUS CALCIUM LEVELS FOUND IN BLOOD

Three major hormones play a complex role in maintaining proper levels of blood calcium. They are the parathyroid hormone (PTH), 1,25-dihydroxyvitamin D (calcitriol) and calcitonin. These hormones act at bone, kidney and small intestine sites to help maintain the proper levels of calcium.

When calcium intake is not adequate, parathyroid hormone production rises and the needed calcium is liberated from the bones. This hormone also boosts absorption of calcium in the small intestine. As soon as blood calcium levels are where they should be, PTH production falls and bone stops being eroded.

These hormones are extremely good at maintaining blood calcium levels within narrow limits. But if these limits are exceeded, as they are in many cancer patients and in people with parathyroid disease, symptoms ranging from mild (loss of appetite, nausea, constipation, abdominal pain, thirst, frequent urination, vomiting) to severe (delirium, confusion, coma, death) can result.

How can this happen? How can levels of calcium rise beyond what is safe? First, let's make clear that eating foods rich in calcium cannot have this effect—*unless you are also consuming calcium mineral salt supplements.*

In the days when ulcers were treated with several glasses of milk per day, plus calcium carbonate antacids, plus sodium bicarbonate (alkali), hypercalcemia was more common. Medicine even had a name for it: "milk-alkali syndrome." Now that ulcer treatments have changed, this is less common; however, with so many Americans swallowing high-dose calcium pills, calcium-containing antacids, glass after glass of milk and tub after tub of yogurt (don't you know it "does a body good?"), it would seem that this syndrome could be resurging. In fact, authorities have set 2,500 mg per day as the top safe intake level of calcium from food plus supplements.

In some people, an overactive parathyroid gland causes too much calcium to remain in the body, instead of being filtered out through the kidneys. This leads to soaring blood calcium levels: a condition known as *parathyroid-mediated hypercalcemia* or just *hyperparathyroidism*. Some cases of this condition are caused by kidney failure or poor kidney function, which spurs the parathyroid gland to make too much of its calcium-preserving hormone. Often called the disease of "stones, bones and abdominal groans," it causes serum calcium levels to soar. The incidence of hyperparathyroidism increases with age.

In the United States, hypercalcemia is a fairly common metabolic emergency. Statistics show that primary hyperparathyroidism occurs in 25 of 100,000 persons in the general population and in 75 per 100,000 people who are hospitalized. In the U.S., more than 50,000 new cases are diagnosed each year.

What's more, the use of calcium mineral salts in high doses has been linked to cardiovascular disease. Studies have found that coronary artery calcium deposits may be an independent risk factor for heart attacks—independent of cholesterol counts and high blood pressure. Other research finds that women who take high doses of calcium salts are at increased risk of heart attacks. Could this be due to high doses of a single nutrient depleting others needed for heart health? You bet. Could it be due to the equivalent of pouring gasoline under your car's hood, hoping enough of it gets in there to start up the engine? This could play a role as well. When you dump all of these highly processed calcium salts into your body—way more than it can effectively process and utilize, in a form it hardly knows what to do with—you're asking for trouble.

You *can* get too much calcium. It isn't too hard to do this. What *is* hard is to get enough of the right kind of calcium—the kind that's essentially predigested by plants.

Because many of the common calcium supplements that people ingest are filled with calcium mineral salts that do more harm than good by increasing blood calcium to dangerous levels, people need to be vigilant in feeding their bodies with whole-food calcium. You can accomplish this with a wide array of delicious calcium-rich foods—foods you might not currently consider as calcium sources—that are easy to prepare. Supplements are available that contain bone-building minerals, herbs and nutrients that support calcium's many vital processes and the body is able to break down because these sources come from . . . food.

All this being said, calcium intake—the **form** you consume and the **amount** you consume—is only part of the Whole Body Bone Building equation. Also requiring consideration: your body's ability to absorb and utilize calcium. Many "calcium-robbers" can have powerful impact here.

Chapter Two

Bone Leachers Contribute to Calcium Crisis

A steady diet of white flour, sugar, and saturated fat will obviously not feed the bones optimal levels of the nutrients they need. Neither will standard calcium supplements. On the other side of the equation, bones can become vulnerable due to what I like to call "bone leachers"—any substance or lifestyle choice that can disrupt the balance of minerals in bones, accelerating loss of bone and reducing bone building. And as is almost always the case with health, any influence that negatively impacts one body system will have negative impacts on others. It follows that improving bone health with proper nutrient balance will improve the health of your heart, your immune system, your nervous system, and your digestive system, too.

These calcium-robbing culprits can come in many forms; over time, they can have a serious negative impact on healthy bones. A dull backache that turns into severe back pain is usually an indication of weak bones (You feel like you are coming unglued. Calcium is the glue that holds the body together!). Losing height is also a clear sign that bones are undernourished and weakening. Spinal deformities can result in a stooped posture, or even a "widow's hump." The problem is that when it gets to this point, serious damage has already taken place and pain can become a constant companion.

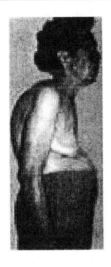
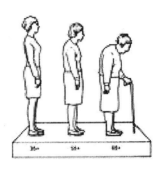

Before bone-leachers begin their harmful calcium-stripping job, we are already losing a good deal of calcium every day through the natural shedding process of the skin, nails, hair, sweat, urine and bowel movements. Because the body cannot make calcium, our bodies are already vulnerable to bone challenges long before bone-leachers swoop in and make the fragility of the situation achingly worse.

How to Build a Dowagers Hump

Think of our bones as the structural frame of our body like the Eiffel Tower somewhat. The many ingredients in the bone has some primary functions: to create these rigid mineralizations (includes the calcium, phosphorous, and other minerals) throughout the bone or to be the glue (the collagen proteins) that holds these mineralized structures within the bone. With someone delevoping a dowagers hump, their spine accumulates tiny fractures due to poor ingredients and lack of weight bearing exercise usually, thus resulting in a stooped, often painful posture. We forget that our bone is very much alive and needs nourishment daily.

Bone-leachers can come from diet induced acidosis (a state where the body has high acidity and low oxygen which is perfect breading ground for disease to develop) from food and drinks, medications, poor exercise habits, lack of sunshine and stress.

DIETARY BONE LEACHERS

As I've already mentioned, Americans have a higher calcium intake than other countries, yet we have the highest incidence of osteoporosis. This "more calcium, more broken bones" paradox is due, in part, to our reliance on dairy and synthetic supplements as sources of calcium rather than a well-balanced, whole-food diet that is rich in calcium and its co-factor nutrients, which are only found in real, live whole foods and regular weight bearing exercise.

Dairy Products

The first bone leacher I'd like to address is . . . dairy. *What?* you might say. *Dairy's supposed to be the BEST source of calcium!* I include this here so prominently due to the fact that we're losing out on daily opportunities to consume plant sources of calcium, because we're so busy gobbling down all this dairy and think we're covered. Here's the hard truth: *rates of osteoporosis are highest in countries where consumption of dairy is highest!*

The dairy industry tells the government—which is responsible for creating dietary recommendations for Americans through the USDA—that they should push dairy as the most important source of dietary calcium. This is not because it's the best source; although milk does contain a higher density of calcium than most other foods, there are many factors that inhibit that calcium's use by the body, and a host of other reasons why we should not suckle from a cow's udder. (We are the only animal that makes the milk of another animal a dietary staple. Plus a calf has 4 stomachs to digest milk—we don't!) It's because they believe that Americans won't really eat that other stuff—those plants, whole grains & legumes that are our true best calcium sources. And it's true that given a choice between a sweetened carton of yogurt or a serving of boiled collard greens, most Americans will choose the dairy delight, hands down. But people should have access to the truth about calcium sources and be allowed to make their own choices when they fully understand the price of making dairy their prime source of calcium. I'll cover this in detail later on, in Chapter 5. It's amazing how powerful advertising can be. I just saw a popular brand of yogurt advertisement saying that ½ the population of women (in the U.S.?-unclear!) lack calcium and vitamin D. They allude to the fact that this yogurt will give you what you need to fix this crisis. Who is there to protect the consumer?

Dietary recommendations made by the government—including the various versions of the Food Pyramid—are tempered strongly by the financial interests of the processed food industry. No one's making big bucks selling collard greens; the big money is made when simple ingredients are highly processed and sold in bags, boxes, and cans. Marion Nestle, Ph.D., M.P.H., author and past chair of the Department of Nutrition at New York University, puts it this way:

> Food is a $1.3 trillion annual business, with the vast percentage of profits going to added-value products rather than basic commodities. It pays to turn wheat into sugared breakfast cereals, or potatoes into chips. Farmers get only a small share—18% or so—of the consumer's food dollar, less for vegetables, fruits, and grains than for meat and dairy. So there is a big incentive to marketers to make food products with cheap raw ingredients like fat and sugar. And they do—to the tune of 12,000 or so new products every year. There are now 320,000 foods on the market; the average large supermarket contains 40,000 to 60,000 food products, more than anyone could possibly need or want. [Handout from S'Cool Food lecture, titled "School Food, Public Policy, and Strategies For Change," also posted at www.foodpolitics.com]

You'll get the full scoop on milk in the chapter that follows this one.

ACID/BASE IMBALANCES

The earliest cells were packets of seawater within stiff cell walls. Seawater has a pH of around 7.5 to 8.4. Neutral pH, where acid and base are balanced, is right around 7.0; below that is acidic, above that is basic (alkaline). Cells have come a long way since then, and they've become vastly more complex and differentiated. They've developed their very own miniscule organ systems (*organelles*) and they have developed complex chemical reactions involving proteins and enzymes.

Living cells have strict control over pH levels, because even the slightest push above or below the range compatible with life will lead to the cell's demise. Optimal pH in the human body is right around 7.41. If pH rises above 7.42 (becomes too alkaline) or falls below 7.38 (becomes too acidic), proteins are rendered unable to function and are digested by the body. Enzymes, which are charged with helping to drive every chemical reaction in the cells of the body, grind to a halt.

True healing of chronic health challenges (including healing bones) occurs only when and if the blood is restored to a normal to slightly alkalinized pH.

Acidosis is vastly more common than alkalosis, and can be *metabolic* (due to problems with the functioning of the body's mechanisms for maintaining acid-base balance; more subtle metabolic acidosis can occur due to poor diet choices) or *respiratory* (due to breathing problems such as asthma or emphysema). Respiratory acidosis is caused by rising carbon dioxide levels in the body. Carbon dioxide is also termed *respiratory acid*. Asthmatics have trouble blowing off enough carbon dioxide to stay at the low end of the acid-base threshold. They can go on for years, even decades, in this state of low-grade acidosis—and this most definitely affects their energy and well-being.

Within the life-or-death pH range, there is some wiggle room. We can use diet to push pH to the low side of normal. Our dietary deficiencies also create an internal environment that forces the body to go into a state of chronic, low-grade metabolic acidosis. This acidosis is brought about by the effect of commonly eaten foods on the acid-base balance of the body, producing an excess of acids in the body and a deficiency of the nutrients that balance acid naturally. Our diets have led to a chronic state of acidosis, in which we have high acidity and low oxygenation in our bodies. This is the perfect breeding ground for "dis-ease" to develop and grow. So when our pH is off, oxygen delivery to cells is reduced (a major cause of the disease process), pathogens form in the blood and can even become pleomorphic-thus changing their shape, mutating, multiplying and also mirroring pathogenicity. Poor pH also causes enzymes that were once "constructive" to become "destructive." The importance of this pH research is so monumental to those fighting any disease, chronically ill, not feeling well or trying to overcome their health challenge(s).

I always ask, "If you put a bone in a vat of acid, what would happen?" It would eat it up (similar to what happens when people drink those dark colas or eat acid forming foods)—right?! It's no wonder we have so many hip and knee replacements!

BONES ON "PLANT RICH" FOODS & BONES ON "ACID FORMING" FOODS

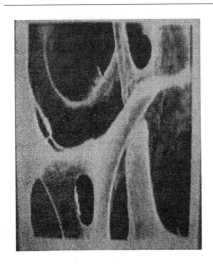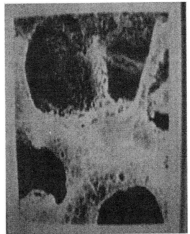

Anthropologists have found little evidence of osteoporosis in aged bones. Our most distant ancestors ate a plant-rich diet that supported a perfect balance between acidic and acid-neutralizing nutrients. The typical modern Western diet, which has only been around for a few decades, is about as different from the prehistoric human's diet as you can get while still calling the stuff consumed "food." It favors protein, which is acid-forming in the body; in fact, modern protein intakes in Western nations are twice what's required for good health. Add to this abundant white bread, sugar, processed food, and salt, all of which tip acid-base balance towards the acidic end. And consider that this diet includes precious few foods rich in potassium and magnesium, both of which are essential for generating *bicarbonate*—the key detoxifying compound used to remove metabolic acids from the body. (See www.cancerfungus.com). Certain medications, environmental pollutants, stress and insufficient sunlight are also triggers in tipping pH balance just enough towards acidity to exert harmful effects on bone, as well as on overall health and well-being.

CAUSES OF BONE LOSS		
Acid Forming Diet	Bone Depleting Medications	Depleted Foods
Environmental Pollutants	Hormone Imbalance	Inactivity
Insufficient Sunlight	pH Imbalance	Stress

In its constant striving towards pH balance, the body looks first to draw calcium from the bloodstream. When it's not available there, the cells then begin to draw from the deep well of alkaline reserves held in the bone—what I call the "bone bank." The deficit in this bank is greater than the U.S. national deficit. We are withdrawing more minerals than we are putting in, which can lead to a state of chronic acidosis, which in turn can lead to a state of low oxygenation. Once again, this kind of acid, hypoxic environment is where most disease thrives.

Getting back to a normal, balanced acid-base status is simple:

1.) Stay away from the big bone-robbers: dark sodas, coffees, excess protein, excess dairy, bone robbing medications, bad fats, bad sugars, and excess sodium.

2.) Aim for a healthy mix of acid and alkaline foods and get active—MOVE & STRENGTHEN YOUR BODY'S!

The big bone-robbers—the top food leaching culprits—are:

Cola-based sodas

A recent study featured in the *American Journal of Clinical Nutrition* found that diet and regular colas (dark sodas like Pepsi, Dr. Pepper, and Coke) have a direct impact on bone loss in women. Researchers looked at 1,413 women and 1,125 men, ages 29 to 86 and found a *significant loss of bone density* in the women—but not men—who drank colas. Green tea, super foods, or water would be a much better choice for beverages.

Investigators at Tufts University found that women who drank three or more colas a day had four percent lower bone mineral density than those who did not drink these sodas. Why would sodas erode bone? Some believe it's the high content of phosphoric acid in these beverages. We need phosphorus to build bone, but if you're taking in huge amounts in sodas every day, your intake of this mineral is out of balance with your intake of calcium—and this can lead to bone loss. A continued low pH that comes from these dark sodas is a pH that is close to death.

Excess protein

> *Eating a high-protein diet is like pouring acid rain on your bones.*
>
> —JOHN McDOUGALL, M.D.,
> of the Physicians' Committee for Responsible Medicine

Protein is essential for energy, muscle, and a sharp mind. Lack of dietary protein is a massive problem on the global scale; in many parts of the world, *kwashiorkor*—protein malnutrition—robs millions of proper growth and even of their lives each year. In the U.S. and other Western nations, however, it's a different story. This is particularly true in the thick of the new resurgence of high-protein, low-carbchydrate diets.

The body only requires just over seven grams of protein per 20 pounds, or 0.8 grams per kilogram of body weight, per day. The average 150-pound adult requires about 50 grams of daily protein; the human body can handle 40–60 grams of protein per day. According to a large survey published by the National Academies Press involving thousands of people who gave dietary information, Westerners consume protein well in excess of these recommendations. (Check out the data from the 2005 study, which I've supplied in the table in the back)

Amino acids, which are the building blocks of protein, are acid-forming when broken down. High protein intake causes the kidneys to filter more calcium out of the bloodstream and far less of that calcium to be reabsorbed into the circulation, where it is accessible for bone building. More of that calcium is drained out of the body in the urine. A higher protein intake may weaken bones because the digestion and elimination of protein by-products can make your body more acidic.

I suggest that you avoid red meat altogether and meet your protein needs by eating heart-friendly vegetarian sources such as whole grains, beans and peas as well as omega-3 fatty acid-rich fish such as salmon. The super grain quinoa is not only highly absorbable and usable to the body, but it is the richest grain source of complete protein with all the essential amino acids and *without* the acid! It also happens to be rich in calcium! In the Women's Health Study, which involves several hundred thousand women being tracked over decades, women whose dietary records indicated that they consumed 95 or more grams of protein per day had a 20 percent higher

chance of breaking a wrist than women who consumed 68 grams
of protein per day or less.

Average Protein Intakes for Different Age Groups in the U.S., 2005

Age	Protein intake (grams) for boys and men	Protein intake (grams) for girls and women
9–13	79.1	65.3
14–18	99.0	66.5
19–30	104	63.3
31–50	99.4	64.9
51–70	86.8	61.7

From Dietary Reference Intakes for Energy, Carbohydrate, Fiber, Fat, Fatty Acids, Cholesterol,
Protein, and Amino Acids (Macronutrients), 2005, The National Academies Press, http://
books.nap.edu/openbook.php?record_id=10490&page=1060

Inadequate protein

All things considered, bone-building requires adequate dietary protein. The matrix of bone can't be constructed with appropriate mass
and density without it. Although *inadequate* protein can present
problems when it comes to maintaining optimal bone mass and
preventing osteoporosis, this is rarely an issue except in elderly people over the age of 70—the only Americans, it appears, who tend to
eat too little protein.

Eating steaks and chicken and eggs by the dozen won't help
much at that point. The National Academies Press surveys do show
that American children eat enough protein to build strong bones.
Any child that doesn't consume enough protein for his or her age
and size will need to be encouraged to consume more. Once protein needs are met—perhaps an egg in the morning or a hemp protein shake, a nut butter sandwich at lunch, and a three-ounce piece
of fish (see the chipotle salmon cakes in the recipe section), an in-
credible bone building salad (see recipe section) or quinoa salad at
dinner will do the trick—a diet abundant in plants rich in calcium

and other vital minerals is adequate to build powerful bones without the acid forming and calcium leaching effects.

Too much sodium—The "wrong salt"

Skipping the salt shaker is a great way to protect your bones. Typical table salt or sodium encourages your body to excrete more calcium through urination and sweating. Even if you never pick up a salt shaker, it is imperative that you read food labels carefully. Many packaged and processed foods have extremely high levels of added sodium for flavor. The type of sodium or salt our body actually *needs* to maintain the proper sodium to potassium ratio inside and outside the cells is rich in minerals and has not been processed. You may have seen Celtic Salt or Sea Salt that maintains the minerals (especially iodine) from the water it is taken from. These minerals are much utilized and needed to the human body as we said before—our cell content was once very close to "little oceans" in composition.

> ### THE "RIGHT" SALT
>
> When you do use salt—and one teaspoon a day is plenty—be sure to choose sea salt instead of iodized table salt (sodium chloride). Sea salt naturally contains complementary minerals that enable your body to better process the sodium it contains as well as natural support for your thyroid.

The general rule is that we need just one teaspoon of the good Sea or Celtic salt daily. Any more of the processed, denatured sodium, can be detrimental to bone health. It's best to get rid of that source from your cupboards all together.

Knowing which of the foods listed on the next page are bone-leaching and which are bone-preserving is half the battle (www.radiantgreens.com or www.energyessentials,com). Cutting bone leachers out of your diet or eating them in moderation make up the other half of the equation of maintaining strong bones via dietary interventions. It's best to keep the 80–20 Rule. Use 80% alkaline forming foods and 20% acid forming foods in your daily food choices. (Refer to www.curesinthekitchen.com for recipes, food lists and other great resources).

Acid-Forming and Alkaline-Forming Foods

The acid-forming or alkaline nature of a food is determined by its effect on the pH of urine. Urine pH can vary from a very basic 4.5 to a very acidic 8. An acidic food will cause urine pH to fall, while alkaline food will bring urine pH higher.

Acid-forming (bone-leaching) foods	Alkaline (bone-saving) foods
Meats (especially organ meats)	Mineral water
Broths made from bones and other animal parts	Most fruits
Sour cream	Most vegetables
Aged cheeses	*Especially:*
Fermented foods (such as wine, sauerkraut and miso)	Oranges
	Yams
Fish	Potatoes
Milk	Spinach and other leafy
greens	Zucchini
Cheese	Watermelon
Chocolate	Carrots
Eggs	Bananas
Soy	Broccoli
Yogurt	Onions
Beans	Grape juice
Poultry	Lemon juice
Most grains	Red wine

PHARMACEUTICAL BONE LEACHERS

Practitioners of Traditional Chinese Medicine (TCM) have long looked for the cause of an illness rather than treating just the symptoms. So have other traditional forms of medicine that have been around far longer than modern, allopathic Western drug-based, symptom-squelching, wait-to-make-a-change-until-you're-really-sick medicine.

The idea behind TCM and other traditional medical practices is that you can reverse a disease process long before you're felled by it.

Practitioners of these ancient healing arts know how to read patients' subtle signs of imbalance, and how to prescribe just the right changes in every aspect of the patient's life—diet, supplements, herbs, exercise, stress coping mechanisms, relationships, the whole ball of wax—to re-balance the body into its most perfect working order. And let's face it—much of the time, we don't really need any medical practitioner to tell us that we're out of balance, or that perhaps we shouldn't eat fast food and drink *molto grande* sweetened coffee drinks every day. It's just hard to have the discipline to make the appropriate changes.

Popping over-the-counter or prescription pills to try to subdue symptoms is the norm in Western medicine. It's such a habit now to swallow a drug for every ill that we often don't recognize that doing so is always an equation with both risks and benefits . . . and that the risks can be extreme.

This Western approach to disease, I'm certain, is contributing to compounding health challenges—both from neglect of a fundamental imbalance in diet or lifestyle and from terrifying side effects of highly potent medications. These side effects, all too often, end up mistaken as a progression of the disease process . . . and medicated with additional drugs! Another risk to consider here: that you're just quelling a symptom—your body's cry for help—rather than seeking to understand and deal with the root problem.

I do understand that some people rely on drugs to live a more comfortable life or need certain medications to prevent health catastrophes. But, as a whole, I believe we've gone overboard on prescription drugs.

Loss of calcium from bone is a side effect of multiple prescription drugs. Most of these drugs are used long-term, over a period of years or decades, to treat chronic medical conditions—setting the user up for osteoporosis as he or she ages. Drugs given to people with rheumatoid arthritis, asthma, hypothyroidism (low thyroid hormone activity), seizures, and gastrointestinal diseases (including heartburn, gastro esophageal reflux disease or GERD, and inflammatory bowel diseases like Crohn's disease) have side effects that can damage bones by leaching away at the calcium in our bones.

In fact, a news story by ABC (2007) found that popular prescription heartburn medications taken for a year or more can significantly raise the risk of a broken hip in people over 50 years old. When you quench stomach acids with antacids, proton pump inhibitors or H2 blocker drugs, the body is less able to absorb calcium and other minerals from the foods you eat. What's very disturbing is that these antacids are marketed to kids like they are candy to cure their tummy ills while their poor diet continues. Is it no wonder that these kids bone breaks have increased so dramatically?!

This heartburn medication news alert is alarming, because "the general perception is they are relatively harmless," said Dr. Yu-Xiao Yang, study co-author of the University Of Pennsylvania School Of Medicine. Many of these medicines that were once only available by prescription are, today, easily purchased over-the-counter by people who pop them like candy to control heartburn—even as they continue to indulge in foods and lifestyle choices that make the problem worse.

Bone-Robbing Medications

All of these drugs deplete calcium from the body in some way, increasing risk of osteoporosis.

Type of Medication	What It Treats	Other Details Worth Knowing
Antidepressants (Prozac, Zoloft, Celexa, Luvox, Paxil, Effexor, Lexapro)	Depression, anxiety.	Studies show increased risk of bone fracture with long-term use of popular antidepressant medications.
Anticonvulsants (Cilontin, Dilantin)	Seizures.	Also used to treat depression, bipolar disorder, chronic pain.
Barbiturates (phenobarbitol, secobarbitol, amobarbitol)	Pain.	Highly addictive; rarely used since newer pain medications are less risky.

Glucocorticoids, also known as steroid drugs (prednisone, prednisolone, methylprednisone)	Excess inflammation, asthma, autoimmune diseases like Crohn's disease, lupus, and rheumatoid arthritis.	Even inhaled steroids used to treat asthma (such as fludrocortisone acetate and beclometasone) can eat away at the skeleton over time.
Digoxin	To regulate an irregular heartbeat or treat heart failure	Only used when no other medications solve the problem.
Estrogen/progestin hormone replacement therapy (Prempro and others)	Treating menopause symptoms such as hot flashes.	Estrogen is a hormone produced by the ovaries; it does help to protect against bone loss once menopause occurs and the ovaries stop most of their production of estrogen. Many physicians still prescribe estrogen replacement to slow bone loss. CAUTION: These replacement therapies come with high risks, including increased risk of breast cancer and blood clots, and should be very carefully considered. For more on menopause and bone health, please see Chapter 4 on the menopausal bone connection.

Oral contraceptives	Birth control and regulation of difficult periods.	The birth control pill delivers a steady stream of estrogen, which is in contrast to the surges that occur in the body off the pill. Keep in mind: **It is the *surges* of estrogen that aids in strong bone formation.**
Gonadotropin releasing hormones (GnRH)	Endometriosis.	This disease has been linked with high estrogen levels, and has been successfully treated with the use of *natural* progesterone, estrogen's balancing hormone that is made in the ovaries each month. For more, see John Lee, M.D. and Virginia Hopkins' book, *Hormone Balance Made Simple* (Wellness Central, 2006). You'll find out more on endometriosis below.
Cyclosporine A	Prescribed as an immunosuppressive drug, usually for rheumatoid arthritis (RA).	Rheumatoid arthritis has been found to respond well to gluten-free, dairy-free, vegetarian and vegan diets, as well as periodic fasting and the "paleo" diet (meat, vegetables, and little else). Milk and gluten-containing

		grains have been found, in several studies, to worsen RA symptoms.
Loop diuretics (Lasix, Burinex, Torem)	High blood pressure.	High blood pressure responds remarkably well to dietary changes, exercise, and stress relief measures. **It's ironic that calcium, which is so important for maintaining proper blood pressure, is drained by these commonly used anti-hypertensive drugs.**
Potassium-sparing diuretics (amiloride, spironolactone, triamterene)	High blood pressure.	
Heparin	A blood thinner used to prevent heart attack and stroke.	Vitamin E, garlic, fish oil: all are natural blood thinners. You can talk to your doctor about these alternatives if you are interested in stopping this drug.
Bile acid sequestrants (cholestyramine, colestipol)	Used to lower high blood cholesterol levels.	These are older drugs that have mostly been replaced by the statins, such as Zocor, Lipitor, Mevacor, and Crestor—alternatives that don't deplete calcium, although they do deplete another nutrient called coenzyme Q10 that's essential for heart health.

See www.energyessentials.com for liver cleansing information.

Some people rely on prescription drugs for survival or for enhanced quality of life, but most of those who think they're dependent could potentially wean themselves off with the right dietary and lifestyle shifts. They don't make the effort because they aren't clear about the risks of even the most commonly prescribed prescription drugs. I was at a health trade show not long ago and met a couple who were on 28 different drugs between the two of them. They were desperate to reduce and eliminate as many as possible but were in fear because the side effects were so awful. They said they felt like they consumed more pills than food in a day. This is a sad reality for a large population in the U.S. Fortunately, they have found natural alternatives and are dealing with the cause, rather than the effect. They have reduced their prescription drug intake by over half with the help of their health care provider.

Every synthetic, chemical drug lacks the wisdom to truly collaborate and cooperate with your body. They are all toxic to some extent. Whole foods and whole food nutrients have powerful medicinal qualities that work in far better concert with the body. They were made to cleanse, strengthen, nourish, nurture & help heal and rejuvenate on a cellular level. Our cells make up every organ and gland, vein & artery, bone, tissue, and muscle in our body. Nature has much more strength and "plant intelligence" to heal than any pharmaceutical, and more money needs to be spent to research these kinds of solutions and their benefits.

Do some research to see whether a practitioner of alternative medicine (for example, a naturopathic physician) or practitioner of traditional medicine (such as a TCM practitioner or Ayurvedic physician) has suggestions for you that might help you reduce your use of medication. Don't assume a drug is safe because it's FDA-approved or because you saw an ad for it on TV. The top motive of pharmaceutical companies is profit, not people, and their marketing and research and development efforts are all about getting as many people on as many drugs as possible for as long as possible. Once again, it's amazing that people will actually take a drug that has so many serious side effects that could potentially even kill them. Yep—as author, Dr. Tony O'Donnell says, "If you don't have plan for your life—you will fit in to someone else's."

If you conclude that you do, indeed, require any of these medicines, discuss your situation with your doctor to find out if these drugs are putting you at risk for osteoporosis—especially if you are post-menopausal, or have a family history of bone disease. Give it the thought it needs—as if *your life depended on it*. Because it just might.

OTHER "BONE-ROBBERS" TO BE WARY OF

Synthetic nutritional supplements, excessive stress, and lack of physical activity can contribute to bone loss. So can certain disease processes.

Iron supplements

If you use an iron supplement, it is crucial that you don't take it at the same time as your calcium supplement. Most forms of calcium can interfere with the absorption of iron. Whole-food sources of vitamin C—including Peruvian camu camu fruit, gogi berries, pomegranate juice (www.radiantgreens.com), black currant, ascerola cherry—can override this calcium-blocking effect.

Iron deficiency is a major problem worldwide. Some estimates put the number of iron-deficient people on the planet at *four to five billion*. The standard tests used to test for iron deficiency don't adequately detect it, and B12 supplements, which are quite popular nowadays, can actually worsen iron deficiency as it drives the iron count down if it is already low. Restless legs syndrome, a brand-new diagnosis that has hit epidemic proportions, is believed by some experts to be caused by iron deficiency. Make sure your doctor tests your serum ferritin levels to determine your iron counts.

Women who are still menstruating are more likely to end up iron deficient. If you choose to take an iron supplement, avoid ferrous oxide and other "industrial," chemical, non-plant-derived forms of iron. Choose instead plant-based forms of iron, which contain abundant co-factors and is well-utilized by the body. The body takes what it needs and any excess is released as opposed to heme iron from meat, which can overload the body and lead to serious health challenges. (See references in the back).

Lack of vitamin D

Vitamin D deficiency is another major silent epidemic whose time has come to expose. It has long been known that vitamin D is crucial for healthy bones. The presence of vitamin D in the small intestine aids in the absorption and calcification of dietary calcium. People with vitamin D deficiency are able to absorb only a third to half as much calcium as those with sufficient levels.

The two most known diseases traditionally associated with severe vitamin D deficiency are rickets in children and osteomalacia in adults—both of which are characterized by a softening or deformation of bone. Chronic vitamin D deficiency is strongly linked to loss of bone density and a higher risk of fractures.

Strangely enough, vitamin D deficiency did not become a health challenge issue until the industrial revolution occurred in the early 1900's. Due to the reduced exposure to the sun as people spent more time inside working and less time out in the sunshine. Sunshine is the most important source of this vitamin as the skin synthesizes the sunlight exposure.

There has been intense scrutiny regarding whether the federal guidelines for Vitamin D are dangerously low leaving millions of people susceptible to serious diseases like cancer, diabetes, heart disease to name a few.

There are numerous studies showing evidence that low levels of vitamin D make men more likely to have heart attacks, kidney disease victims more likely to die, colon & breast cancer victims less likely to survive, and children more likely to develop diabetes. Other studies suggested that higher Vitamin D levels reduce the risk of dying prematurely from any cause. "The bottom line is we now recognize that vitamin D is important for health for both children and adults and may help prevent many serious chronic diseases," said Michael F. Holick, a Professor of Medicine, Physiology and Biophysics at Boston University. Vitamin D offers many health benefits, protection from infectious diseases like tuberculosis and the flu, perhaps mental illnesses including schizophrenia and depression, potentially protecting against heart disease, immune system disorders such as multiple sclerosis and rheumatoid arthritis and multiple forms of cancer.

"Vitamin D has a global effect on many systems," said Bruce Hollis, a Professor of Pediatrics, Biochemistry and Molecular Biology at the Medical University of South Carolina.

While today we are seeing daily amounts of Vitamin D rising from 250 IU's to 400 to even 600 IU's, in the early 1900's, **the amounts** of Vitamin D were much higher In recent years, such highly respected journals as the *American Journal of Clinical Nutrition* have published studies suggesting that 800 or even 1,000 IU of vitamin D is inadequate for osteoporosis prevention. Up to 10,000 IU per day is being recommended for healthy adults—well beyond the supposed "safe limits" established earlier. This particular study was a meta-analysis of 18 clinical trials on vitamin D, involving 57,311 participants. Those who took 300 to 2,000 IU of vitamin D in these trials had a seven percent overall reduction in mortality (risk of death from any cause). Trends towards more significant reduction of mortality were seen in studies lasting longer than three years. It's obvious from the early 1900's information, that miniscule IU's are grossly inadequate compared to the needed milligrams that could change disease as we know it.

"The first thing we'd see is a reduction by 80 % in the incidence of Type 1 diabetes," said Cedric Garland, a Professor of Family and Preventive Medicine at the University of California at San Diego. "The next thing we'd see is a reduction by about 75 percent of all invasive cancers combined, as well as similar reductions in colon cancer and breast cancer, and probably about a 25 percent reduction in ovarian cancer."

Vitamin D adequacy also seems to be important for both breast cancer prevention and survival. A 2008 study revealed a strong link between vitamin D levels in women's bodies and their risk of breast cancer death. Of a large group of women who were diagnosed with breast cancer, only 24 percent were *not* vitamin D deficient at diagnosis. Ten years following diagnosis, 83 percent of those with adequate vitamin D levels at diagnosis were still alive; 79 percent of those with insufficient D levels at diagnosis were still alive; and of those who were frankly *deficient* at diagnosis, only 69 percent were still alive. This adds up to a 73 percent increased risk of death within 10 years of diagnosis in those who were vitamin D deficient.

Low Vitamin D levels have also been linked to increased risk of skin, colon, and prostate cancers, and with depression, bipolar disorder, unexplained musculoskeletal pain, and schizophrenia. You'll learn more about Vitamin D and how to ensure you're getting enough, in Chapter 5.

Lack of weight-bearing exercise

Without a regular exercise routine, you're leaving your body vulnerable to bone loss. There's no way around it! Without exercise, your posture, balance and flexibility become less fine-tuned and you become more prone to falls that can break fragile bones. Unless you engage in consistent weight-bearing activities, you are paving the way for onset of osteoporosis.

The popular belief is that exercise may be too little, too late in someone who has already been losing bone for years—i.e., women who are through the menopausal transition. Maintaining current bone mass may not seem like enough in this case. But the truth is that you *can* build bone, even if you're a menopausal woman . . . even if you're in your 70s, 80s, or beyond! At least two meta-analyses—where researchers gather many studies on the same topic and combine all the data to get the big picture—have found that walking and resistance training both *increase* bone mineral density in women following menopause. This occurs at some of the most vulnerable spots: the hip, the lower spine, and the upper thigh where it enters the hip socket.

If regular workouts build bone even in this most fracture-vulnerable population, imagine how much it will benefit people who are younger, or who are male. It's never too late to get started, and it could make the difference between a terribly painful, bedridden decline in your 70s and a vibrant extra decade of active living. Make sure you start the "Whole Body Bone Building Exercise Program" in Chapter 6 as soon as your health care practitioner says it is o.k. It takes as little as 15 to 20 minutes a day (3 to 4 times a week) and makes you feel better, stronger and rejuvenated right away.

Stress wreaks havoc

We hear a lot about stress these days, and about the damage it might be doing to us internally. People are turning to meditation, yoga and even prescription drugs to handle the heart-pounding, high-anxiety feelings that accompany a stressful situation. So, what really happens to our bodies when we are faced with the flood of fight-or-flight stress hormones that occur when we are under stress?

According to Dr. Lynne Tan of Montefiore Medical Center in New York City, "Stress is a burst of energy. It's our body telling us what we need to do." (Weaver 2006). When the brain detects physical or psychological stress, it releases hormones such as cortisol and neurotransmitters such as adrenaline (epinephrine) and norepinephrine throughout the body. As a result, the heart pumps faster, blood pressure soars, blood sugar elevates and the senses become as sharp as a tack.

Emerging research is showing some upsides to moderate amounts of stress. The hormonal surge and neurotransmitter shift promotes the ability to perform tasks more efficiently, setting the brain and body buzzing. The positive results of "good stress" include a feeling of control, brain cells working at peak capacity, improved heart function and an enhanced immune system, which actually helps the body to ward off infections. A recent study demonstrated that stress could help lower the risk of breast cancer because it curbs the production of estrogen (Weaver 2006).

However, when a person is faced with chronic or severe stress that allows the stress-hormone flood of hormones to be maintained for more than 24 hours, the body faces peril. It may take the form of elevated blood pressure, heart disease, and an overall feeling of fatigue and depression as the adrenals—the source of cortisol—are tapped out.

Signs of too much stress include frequent colds, mental sluggishness, and flare-ups of arthritis and inflammatory bowel disease. As with too much of any good thing, stress can kill. "Over time, if you're constantly in fight or flight, if your heart muscles and valves are awash in the epinephrine, it causes changes in the arteries and in the way that cells are able to regenerate," says Dr. Tan (Weaver 2006).

Life is stressful; there is no way around it. Your techniques for managing the stress, and your attitudes towards it, are key. Dr. Tan tells us that we should "focus the energy like a laser beam on what you need to do . . . Take the extra stress energy . . . and make it into a high-energy, positive situation."

Successfully managing stress can help the body remain in balance—and the balance between bone building and bone breakdown is no exception to this rule. You can use herbs like jujube (also known as Chinese date or red date), astragalus, lemon balm, peoria, chamomile, and valerian to help control stress without addictive pharmaceutical stress-reducers. L-theanine, derived from tea, has potent but not sleepiness-inducing relaxant effects.

Both vitamin C and the B vitamins are depleted by excess, chronic stress. By using a supplemental real vitamin C and B vitamin complex—from whole foods, not isolated USP vitamins—you can promote your body's natural defenses against stress-induced damage and to protect from adrenal burnout. Real food sources of Vitamin C & B complex are like the oil in a car that make the car run-if it is out of oil, the car doesn't run. Vitamin B & C are similar to that with the adrenals-they will run on empty and the hormone levels like cortisol go off the charts and effect the pancreas, throwing off the sugars (often turning to fat and effecting the heart) as well as the thyroid (weight gain, temperature irregularities of too cold or too hot). (see www.energyessentials.com for whole food sources)

High blood sugar, low blood sugar, and your bones

Osteoporosis is considered to be a slow-onset disease, but some intriguing research suggests that it may set in rapidly under certain circumstances. Rapid onset of bone loss appears related to quick cycling of very low blood sugar (hypoglycemia) and high blood sugar (hyperglycemia).

To understand how this happens, you'll need to grasp the basics of insulin resistance and diabetes. The scale of these problems is enormous today. Obesity, cardiovascular disease, high blood fats, and high cholesterol are all linked with blood sugars that rise too high and stay high. In 2002, at least 54 million American adults had *impaired glucose tolerance,* a pre-diabetic state of chronically high blood sugar that almost always leads to developing full-blown diabetes.

Why does this jump in blood sugars happen? The usual source of the problem is a diet high in sugars and refined carbohydrates. Eating a meal high in these ingredients causes blood sugars to rise quickly as the simple carbohydrates they contain are rapidly absorbed into the bloodstream through the intestinal wall. Next, the pancreas—a small organ located at the top of the small intestine—is signaled to crank out the hormone insulin, which escorts all of those sugar molecules into cells, where they can be burned for energy. A quick rise in blood sugar means a quick rise in insulin, which means a quick clearance of sugars from the bloodstream. Now, you've got *hypoglycemia,* and you're craving that next hit of simple carbohydrates. As soon as you get some down your throat, the cycle begins anew.

Along this roller-coaster ride, you're pretty much guaranteed to gain weight, since this cycle makes over consumption of calories more or less impossible to avoid. As the excess pounds pile on, the body eventually tries to stop the madness by becoming *insulin resistant.* They begin to become deaf to the signals of insulin to let sugars inside the cells. At first, the pancreas doesn't want to cooperate, and it cranks out more and more insulin to try to overcome this resistance. This may work for a while, but then you've got a continuing unhealthy cycle of hypoglycemia and hyperglycemia, with high levels of insulin to boot. Both high blood sugars and high insulin are damaging to blood vessels, which is why pre-diabetes and diabetes are linked with drastically increased risk of heart attack, blindness, kidney disease, and nerve damage.

Often, the body does a good enough job at maintaining a workable (but not healthful) balance that symptoms are averted. The person might only have lack of energy and carbohydrate cravings to warn him or her that diabetes is just around the corner.

If this process continues uninterrupted, eventually the pancreas loses steam and can no longer keep up with the demand for evergreater insulin secretion. It becomes exhausted. At that point, blood sugars rise and don't descend. Serious symptoms of diabetes may emerge: extreme thirst, a great deal of urination, extreme hunger, unusual weight loss, extreme fatigue, blurry vision, and irritability. Left untended to, diabetes kills in very short order.

So . . . what's the link to bone health? Low blood sugar triggers production of the stress hormones cortisol and adrenaline—an attempt by the body to normalize blood sugar levels after they have dropped very rapidly. This is one reason why eating sugar and refined flour makes you a little "high," jittery, and irritable. These hormones have *catabolic,* or breaking-down, effects. Repeated bouts of high blood sugar over years has a breaking-down effect on bone and connective tissue. At the height of pre-diabetic hyperglycemic/hypoglycemic cycling, bone loss can be substantial even over the course of a single year.

Breathing shallowly or incompletely

Right now, check in with your breathing. Don't change it; just turn your attention to it. Is it shallow and short? Are you failing to exhale and inhale fully and easily, your chest, abdomen, and ribs moving with the breath? Do you tend to hold your breath or breathe shallowly, particularly when stressed?

If you answered "yes" to all of these questions, you may have yet another lesser-known risk factor for bone loss: *respiratory acidosis.*

Most simply, respiratory acidosis can be described as too much carbon dioxide (CO_2) and not enough oxygen. As a result, the whole body moves towards the acidic side of ideal pH. Breathing in too much air and not exhaling enough of it will cause low-grade respiratory acidosis. At its worst, respiratory acidosis can kill; this is what happens with asthmatics. And knowing what you know now about acid-base balance, you know that in order to neutralize excess acids, your body pulls minerals from the bones.

A friend told me about a yoga workshop she attended where they performed a breath exercise called *holotropic breath work*. This involves self-imposed "heavy breathing" through the mouth, rapidly, to the beat of loud music. "Right away, as the teacher had warned us, our hands and feet cramped up . . . they wouldn't un-cramp. It was excruciating," she told me. "I got pins and needles, I was totally dizzy and anxious . . . when I had to get up in the middle to go to the restroom, I had to be literally guided by one arm—I could barely stand up." Then why do people do this, if it feels so bad? "Some people have a really ecstatic experience," she told me. "They go into states of altered consciousness, have visions and release big emotions . . . the teacher said that *sometimes* it's ecstatic . . . and sometimes it's awful."

This kind of breath work reverses the CO_2/O_2 balance, so that more CO_2 is blown off and more oxygen comes in. It alkalizes the body to an extreme that can be uncomfortable. But with conscious, relaxed, deep, steady breathing throughout the day, you can more gently alkalinize the body in a way that can protect bone. Added benefits: a more regular, relaxed heartbeat (certain heart arrhythmias are linked to poor breathing practices besides a magnesium deficiency) and reduced anxiety.

The best place to learn to breathe properly is in a yoga class. Seek out classes that address *pranayama,* or the yoga of breath, with an experienced instructor. Plenty of DVDs and audio CDs on this type of breath work are available as well.

Diseases that can predispose us to osteoporosis

According to the Surgeon General, some diseases can promote osteoporosis. If you have any of these conditions, it's particularly essential for you to ensure that you are getting adequate bioavailable calcium and the nutrients your body needs to utilize it:

- **Chronic lung disease.** Chronic lung diseases such as asthma, emphysema, sleep apnea or chronic bronchitis create a state of chronic respiratory acidosis, which reduces bone density over time as minerals are pulled from bone to buffer excess acid. One lesser-known way to combat chronic lung problems is to (believe it or not) do a thorough colon cleansing. In traditional medical models, the colon and lungs are sister organs, and when you clear all of the old, stagnant matter out of the colon, lung health is usually improved. The best time for a colon cleanse is in the fall of each year. For more on cleansing and bone health (and overall health too), see the Sidebar.

- **Hyperparathyroidism** is a condition in which the body produces excessive amounts of parathyroid hormone (PTH), which in turn disrupts regulation of calcium. As a result, calcium is taken from the

SEASONAL CLEANSING AND YOUR HEALTH

In the "olden days"—that would be most of human history—we didn't have much choice but to live according to the dictates of the seasons. Then came indoor climate control, electric lights, and global food transit that enable us to get anything we want in any season. In Western nations, we are no longer powerfully affected by temperature, length of day, and seasonal availability of foods. In those olden days, it wasn't unusual to undergo periods of fasting or eating very little during lean seasons, or to have periods of more rest and less activity, or periods of gorging on seasonal plant foods. Most people were also far more physically active and had zero calorie-dense junk food in those days. We consumed fewer calories and burned off more.

To replace these natural fluctuations in an unnatural world, the best solution is seasonal cleansing. In Ayurvedic and Traditional Chinese medicines—two of the oldest, most time-tested traditional medical models on Earth—seasonal cleanses are part and parcel of maintaining health and vitality. These sorts of cleanses gently purge, strengthen, nourish, and rejuvenate our bodies at the cellular level. They allow us to clear our bodies of toxic influences, kick addictions to sugar and other refined carbohydrates, bring blood sugars and hormones into their ideal natural balance, and give the digestive system a much-needed rest.

In fact, the tendency to get sick when seasons change has to do with the body's natural instinct towards self-cleansing.

Stomach flu, head cold, cough—all of these are about concentrating the "yuck" of the past few months and removing it from the body. We can be more proactive about this by cleansing intentionally at the turn of each season. Each organ system is especially responsive at certain times of the year.

Seek out a seasonal cleansing, Traditional Chinese Medicine, or Ayurvedic specialist to help you with these cleanses. Healing retreats involving these kinds of cleanses are offered nationwide. A great book to guide in cleansing is "Miracle Detox Secrets" by Tony O'Donnell, ND, CNC. You can also look at the books of Elson Haas, M.D., a physician who is world-renowned for his expertise on internal cleansing regimens and their

Spring:	liver/gallbladder cleanse
Summer:	heart/small intestine cleanse
Fall:	large intestine/lung cleanse
Winter:	adrenal/kidney/bladder cleanse

benefits: *Staying Healthy With the Seasons* (Celestial Arts, 2003), *Staying Healthy With Nutrition* (Celestial Arts, 2006) and *The New Detox Diet* (Celestial Arts, 2004) or visit an Energy Essentials Cleansing, Weight Loss & Rejuvenation Center near you @ www.energyessentials.com.

bones; blood levels of calcium rise; and increased amounts of calcium may be excreted in urine. This is almost always caused by a benign tumor, which can be surgically removed.

■ **Cancer,** which is any malignant growth or tumor caused by abnormal and uncontrolled cell division that most times has fungus associated with it according to Dr. Tullio Simoncini, M.D. It may spread to other parts of the body through the lymphatic system or the blood stream, and can have detrimental effects on bone. (Google Dr. Tullio Simoncini and candida or sodium bicarbonate)

■ **Chronic hepatic (liver) disease,** which is marked by the gradual destruction of liver tissue over time. Liver disease tends to increase bone breakdown. A whole food & herb liver & gallbladder cleanse and support program is crucial. (see sidebar and references on seasonal cleansing)

■ **Diabetes or impaired glucose tolerance,** which you read about earlier in this chapter.

■ **[Chronic renal (kidney) disease** is the progressive loss of kidney function. The reasons aren't fully understood, but it's believed that poor kidney function creates acidosis in the body, which in turn reduces bone mass as minerals are pulled from the bone to buffer acids. This is why it's so important to do a winter cleanse, which cleanses, strengthens, nourishes, nurtures, and helps heal the kidneys, adrenals, and bladder (see the Sidebar on seasonal cleansing for more on this).

- **Cushing's disease** is also referred to as hyperadrenocorticism— the production of too much adrenal hormone, particularly cortisol. Hyperadrenocorticism occurs for one of two reasons: a tumor of the adrenal gland that produces adrenal hormones, or over-stimulation of the normal adrenal glands from the hormones that control it. Cushing's disease causes increased drinking, increased urination, increased appetite, panting, high blood pressure, and hair loss that is usually evenly distributed on both sides of the body. Other symptoms include a pendulous abdomen, thinning of the skin, calcified lumps in the skin, susceptibility to skin infections and diabetes, and weakening of the bones, heart, nervous system, and skeletal muscles.

- **Multiple sclerosis** (MS) is a chronic degenerative disease of the central nervous system in which gradual destruction of the fatty, conductive myelin sheath around nerves—which is needed to conduct the impulses that control body movements—occurs in patches throughout the brain or spinal cord (or both), interfering with the nerve pathways. MS causes muscular weakness, loss of coordination and speech and visual disturbances. People with MS are at heightened risk of osteoporosis.

- **Rheumatoid arthritis (RA)** occurs when the body's immune system attacks joints, leaving them feeling hot, painful, swollen and often deformed. Internal organs may also be damaged by the disease. A liver and gallbladder cleanse can work wonders for people with RA. (see References in the back of book)

- **Endometriosis is the pres**ence of endometrial tissue (which normally lines the uterus) in abnormal locations such as the ovaries, fallopian tubes and abdominal cavity. It causes pain, heavy periods, and (sometimes) infertility. Recent research has found that most women, when they menstruate, have some cells from the endometrium that "reflux" up into the abdominal cavity; in some women, the immune system reacts to these cells and endometriosis is the result. Heightened levels of a hormone called *interleukin-1* are characteristic in women with endometriosis, and it's believed that this hormone is the link between thinning bones and this disease—a condition that exists in a third of infertile women.

- **Sarcoidosis** involves inflammation that produces tiny lumps of cells in various organs in the body. These tiny lumps can grow and clump together, forming harmful clusters in an organ, negatively impacting its function. Sarcoidosis usually starts in the lungs or lymph nodes and almost always occurs in more than one organ at a time. Signs of this disease may include a disturbed heart rhythm, arthritis in the ankles or vision challenges. In sarcoidosis, calcium metabolism is altered in a way that negatively impacts the bones.

- **Hemochromatosis** is a hereditary metabolic disorder that causes increased absorption of iron. It occurs in about one of every 250 people—those who are unlucky enough to inherit one gene for the condition from each parent. Excess iron is deposited in the body tissues and organs, such as the liver, heart, or pancreas, where it may become toxic. Bones tend to be weakened and risk of osteoporosis is heightened in people with this disorder. Recommended for those with hemochromatosis: a vegetarian or vegan diet. This is because *heme iron* from meat doesn't know how to shut off and gets over loadedand is linked with certain cancers and heart challenges. N*on-heme iron* from plant foods has "plant intelligence" that seems to know where and how much iron is needed and passes what isn't needed right through the body quite easily. Eating plenty of plant foods also helps reduce iron levels in those with iron overload by supplying the body with natural inhibitors of iron absorption, such as phytates.

Since there are no warning signs that the bone-building process is out of balance, it usually doesn't become known until bones become so weak that a sudden strain, bump or fall causes a fracture or a vertebra to collapse. This injury is a direct result of calcium deprivation. Still, many don't make the connection that their bones are *starving* for nutrients. Everyone reading this book and all those you love would do well to make an effort to fill that bone bank way before osteoporosis even has a glimmer of a chance to set in.

So . . . the question remains: how do we optimally feed the bones? How do we engage in prevention? The medical and nutritional mainstream would tell you to drink milk and eat cheese and yogurt; and it would tell you to swallow calcium pills loaded with synthetic calcium, perhaps with a little synthetic vitamin D and magnesium added. These measures fall far short of optimal. Read on to see why and what you can do to properly nourish your bones— starting now.

Chapter Three

Got Calcium?

WHAT YOU NEED TO KNOW ABOUT MILK

In the "Happy Cows" ads created by the California Milk Board, cows lounge in grassy fields or cozily nestle in straw-filled barns, saying witty things to one another. The message: good dairy foods come from happy cows. Happy cows come from California. These ads cost the California Milk Advisory Board some $37 million a year.

Unfortunately, these commercials do *not* reflect the way the vast majority of dairy cows are actually treated. In fact: if animal cruelty laws regarding cows—which are intelligent, social, docile beings, revered by Hindus as a symbol of the giving character of Mother Nature—were the same as those regarding companion animals like cats and dogs, most dairy producers in California and elsewhere in the U.S. would be in big trouble with the law.

The cows who yield calcium-rich dairy in California live packed tightly together in mud, urine, and feces-filled dry feedlots. The word "dry" is actually a misnomer, as the feces and urine these animals stand and lie down in are sometimes cleaned out only twice a year. This so-called dry-lot system was created to eke the maximum output of milk from cows while incurring as little overhead as possible.

Feces and urine are a big problem on these feedlots. California's 1.5 million cows produce over 30 million tons of waste per year. Cow feces have to be disposed of, but while they pile up, they dry out and send particulates into the air, which mix with airborne industrial pollutants and create some of the worst air pollution in the nation. People who live near these big dry-lot dairy farms are at increased risk of asthma and other respiratory problems. A lesser-known problem: cow burps, which scientists from UC Davis say are a major cause of ozone air pollution. All in all, the dairy-farm-rich San Joachin Valley in California has air quality worse than that of Los Angeles.

Nitrogen from cow manure often pollutes groundwater around these farms, leading to algal blooms and fish kills. Killer bacteria also pass into groundwater, and this can end up contaminating crops—a kind of contamination that was believed to be the source of the *e.coli* spinach scare in 2007. People who live around dairy farms also have higher incidence of diarrheal diseases. You may not have heard about the deaths of three low-wage workers who, while performing the unenviable job of maintaining the manure and urine disposal machinery at California dairies, were overcome by methane gas and drowned in pools of liquified cow manure. (To their credit, the "Happy Cows" ads don't try to give us any happy impressions about those who work on or live near dairy farms.)

At any given time, a third of California's dairy cows are suffering from painful udder infections. Half suffer from other illnesses like milk fever, Johne's Diseaes, laminitis, bovine immune deficiency virus, and bovine leukemia virus. Most dairy cattle are dosed up on drugs and hormones that increase milk production, leading many of the cows' udders to swell to enormous proportions. A cow's natural lifespan is 25 years; most of these so-called "happy cows" are sent to the slaughterhouse by the time they are six years old.

To ensure a steady supply of milk, dairy cows are artificially inseminated each year and give birth to a calf, which is immediately taken from its mother. If the calf is male, it is either sent off to a feedlot to be rapidly fattened and slaughtered to yield hamburgers, steaks, and other American food staples, or it may end up chained into a stall so tiny it can't turn around, then slaughtered at 16 weeks of age to yield tender white veal.

What about organically, humanely raised dairy? Of course, this is a better alternative. If you decide to include dairy products in your diet, you and the planet will be better off if you choose dairy from organic, free-range, grass-grazed, humanely treated cows. But you should not rely on any kind of dairy—even if you're bringing it in from Bessie after you've milked her by hand, then turned her loose in your own backyard grassy field—to give your body the calcium it needs to maintain strong bones. And you should not consider milk to be the healthy food it's touted to be by the dairy industry or its government supporters.

Milk is touted as the best bone-strengthening food around. The scientific evidence on this just doesn't add up. Really, the propounding of dairy as an essential food has more to do with economics than it does with actual evidence of health benefits.

Why the gap between image and reality? It all boils down to dollars. In late 2006, Dr. David Ludwig performed a study of the influence of beverage industry money (including that supplied by milk producers and grape juice producers) on the outcome of research studies on those beverages. Not surprisingly, his survey found that studies of beverages were four to eight times more likely to end up showing health benefits for the beverage when funded by companies that make and sell those beverages.

In other words: when milk processors hire a scientist to do a study on the health benefits of dairy, that scientist is four to eight times more likely to end up with a study that supports those health benefits than a researcher who isn't taking milk processors' money to support his or her research.

Pyramid Palaver

The USDA's Food Pyramid, revised every five years, is supposed to reflect the efforts of the nation's best scientific minds to establish workable, practical dietary guidelines for the public. What most of us don't know as we try to make sense of this Pyramid (which becomes more inscrutable with each revision) is that the food and beverage industries intensely lobby the government during each of these revisions.

The National Dairy Council, the Soft Drink Association, the

National Cattlemen's Beef Association, the Wheat Foods Council, and the American Meat Institute are among the powerful lobbying groups that get involved very intimately in this process. They lobby hard even to influence the selection of the nutrition experts who create the Pyramid, and they lobby to ensure that their products are included as prominently as possible in the recommendations of the USDA. The resulting guidelines are always shaped by these lobbying efforts.

The 2006 version of the Food Pyramid—or, more specifically, the "My Pyramid Interactive Food Guidance System"—reflects this industry influence. Contrary to nutrition research's clear understanding that refined flour is bad news for health, the Pyramid says that taking in half of your grains as refined flour is A-OK. Despite what we know about the huge differences between protein sources like beans, red meat, poultry, and fish, and about different nutritional impact from different kinds of oils and fats, the recommendations for protein and added fat are lumped into single categories. And despite strong evidence—which you'll learn about in this chapter—that dairy is not the best source of calcium and that it has health liabilities, this new Pyramid says that you should get three servings of dairy per day.

Sure, we all need to make a living. The dairy industry employs a lot of people. The economy benefits when the dairy deception is supported and people stock up on milk, yogurt, and cheese. But this will come back to bite us eventually—as those who believed that dairy calcium would protect their bones begin to shrink and crumble and the medical system becomes completely overwhelmed with the care of millions of osteoporosis patients.

Milk Does *Not* Do A Body Good— Unless It's Mother's Milk

Fifty years ago, when milk was fresh, untainted, and delivered to our doors in glass bottles; when it had to be consumed right away, before it spoiled—in those days, milk did a body more good than it does today. Back then, cows were free to graze whole foods fresh off the ground. Cows were not dosed up on hormones that encouraged a larger and faster supply of milk. In those simpler times, few things were as delicious or pure as a glass of milk—although that milk was still not an ideal source of calcium, for reasons you'll discover later in this chapter.

Fast-forward to today, post-second millennium. Now, there are many things you should know about that "pure" milk you are giving your children or drinking yourself with the hopes of getting enough calcium into your bones.

If you were lucky, breast milk was your first food and beverage when you entered the world. Mother's milk is all that's required for complete vitamin, mineral, protein, and fatty acid nutrition and a full tummy during the first five to six months of life. A breast-fed baby gets plenty of rich immune-building substances in the bargain, including antibodies and specialized nutrients tailor-made to prepare him or her for the challenges of life. This infusion of health-promoting substances allows infants to thrive in their new worlds.

When our mothers moved us off of the breast and on to cow's milk, we were encouraged to drink lots of it to continue to grow stronger, smarter and bigger. We were told that milk has all the calcium needed for the health of our bones.

The truth is that the calcium found in milk does *very little* for our bones. Without magnesium, milk is not well absorbed or utilized by the skeleton. Cow's milk is *a poor source* of magnesium, a mineral required for bone building, and it contains the wrong balance between calcium and phosphorus for human bone health. Milk that has not received a fat content reduction is rich in saturated fat and cholesterol which contributes to an increased risk of atherosclerosis and coronary heart disease. And it has been linked to increased risk of certain cancers.

CALCIUM, MILK AND OSTEOPOROSIS

The recommendation to drink three glasses of low-fat milk or eat three servings of other dairy products per day to prevent osteoporosis is another step in the wrong direction. . . . Three glasses of

low-fat milk add more than 300 calories a day. This is a real is-
sue for the millions of Americans who are trying to control their
weight. What's more, millions of Americans are lactose intoler-
ant, and even small amounts of milk or dairy products give them
stomachaches, gas, or other problems. This recommendation ig-
nores the lack of evidence for a link between consumption of
dairy products and prevention of osteoporosis. It also ignores the
possible increases in risk of ovarian cancer and prostate cancer
associated with dairy products.

STATEMENT FROM THE HARVARD SCHOOL

OF PUBLIC HEALTH, 2005

We have been conditioned to believe that milk is good for our bones because it is rich in calcium. However, emerging studies do *not* support this belief system. As a nation that gets 75 percent of its calcium from dairy products, this is information that needs to be known and acted upon to reverse the tide of a burgeoning osteoporosis epidemic.

Clearly, calcium from vegetable sources is better absorbed than calcium from dairy. This is probably due, at least in part, to milk's high content of phosphorus—a mineral that blocks calcium absorption and utilization if taken in too high a ratio to calcium—and acid-producing protein. Calcium absorption from milk is about 30 percent; *from vegetable sources, about 40 to 64 percent of calcium is absorbed or more.*

In 2007, a study was published in the *American Journal of Clinical Nutrition* that should have been front-page news. Researchers performed a kind of study called a *meta-analysis*, where they took data from several studies on the same subject and put it all together to try to get the bigger picture. The 12 studies they gathered were all about calcium intake and risk of osteoporotic fractures. A total of about 175,000 individual subjects (people) were included in this analysis. (The more subjects, the more reliable the study's results.) In the end, the results were a huge slam to the whole idea that more calcium is better: not only did those with the highest calcium intake (800 to 1200 milligrams per day) not receive protection against osteoporosis; they had a *64 percent higher risk of fracture* than those who consumed less calcium.

An earlier series of studies from Harvard Medical School involving over 72,000 women found no relationship between dairy or milk consumption and bone mass. These women never used calcium supplements. The researchers found that women who drank two or more glasses of milk per day did not decrease their risk of hip or forearm fractures any more than women who consumed one glass of milk or less per week (Feskanich 1997 and 2003).

Teens are exhorted to consume their three servings of dairy per day to help maximize bone mass in their youth. But a study by University of Pennsylvania researchers, published in the journal *Pediatrics*, found no relationship between calcium intakes of 500 to 1,500 mg per day and stronger bones in teen girls.

Yale University researchers did their own meta-analysis of 34 studies in 16 countries. They chose countries where people consume the most milk, meat, and other non-vegetarian foods, and found—stunningly—that African-Americans, who consume an average of over 1,000 mg of calcium per day, have a nine times higher risk of hip fracture than black South Africans, who consume, on average, less than 200 mg of calcium per day and almost no dairy. Blacks in South Africa consume far less protein than those in the U.S., as well. The study authors surmise that protein overload may be a more likely culprit in osteoporosis than lack of dairy calcium. Other research supports the notion that only in countries where protein intake is too high is there a serious problem with bone loss and osteoporosis. (More on this below.)

In 2000, the *American Journal of Clinical Nutrition* published a review of all research on calcium and bone health performed since 1985. Its conclusion: "If dairy food intakes confer bone health, one might expect this to have been apparent from the 57 outcomes, which included randomized, controlled trials and longitudinal cohort studies involving 645,000 person-years . . . the body of scientific evidence appears inadequate to support a recommendation for daily intake of dairy foods to promote bone health in the general U.S. population."

Even studies funded by the National Dairy Council have failed to demonstrate that dairy calcium protects the bones. In one such study, postmenopausal women drank three eight-ounce glasses of skim milk daily and their bone density was tracked for a period of two years. Then, their bones were compared to those of women matched for age who had not had the three glasses of milk per day (the placebo group). Women in the milk group had been consuming, on average, 1,400 mg of calcium per day—and they lost bone at *twice the rate* of the women in the placebo group! The researchers concluded that it was probably the 30 percent increase in dietary protein seen in the milk drinkers that caused the accelerated bone loss. They then cited 10 other studies that demonstrated similar results.

THE PROTEIN CONNECTION

Milk and dairy products are touted as good sources of protein. As it turns out, the protein in milk may block the benefits of any calcium it contains. University of San Francisco researchers enrolled 9,000 female subjects aged 65 and up and had them fill out detailed diet questionnaires. Those who had the most acid-producing diets had nearly four times as many hip fractures as those with the least acid-producing diets. (Sellmeyer D)

A German study found that for women, high consumption of protein from animal origin is less beneficial in protecting bones than a high vegetable protein intake. The researchers found that a high calcium intake combined with a high ratio of vegetable protein is more protective against osteoporosis than animal protein (Weikert 2005).

Researcher Robert P. Heaney, Ph.D., had similar results with his investigations of protein intake and calcium loss. He found a direct, linear relationship between increasing protein in the diet and calcium loss in the urine. In an article in the *Journal of the American Dietetic Association,* he wrote that "if protein intake is doubled without changing intake of other nutrients, urinary calcium content increases by 50 percent."

The good news for carnivores: taking supplemental calcium and vitamin D appears to offset the loss of bone that seems to occur in people with high-animal-protein diets. A typical study that demonstrates this point followed 342 healthy 65-and-up men and women; they ate a diet averaging 79 grams of protein per day. Those who took 500 mg of calcium a day and 700 IU of complementary nutrient vitamin D were found to have denser, stronger bones at the end of three years than they did at the start.

What sort of calcium did these women take, and what is the optimal source of supplemental calcium and vitamin D? More on this in Chapter 5.

THE LAST NAIL IN DAIRY CALCIUM'S COFFIN: THE CHINA-OXFORD-CORNELL STUDY

The association between the intake of animal protein and fracture rates appears to be as strong as the association between cigarette smoking and lung cancer.

—COLIN CAMPBELL, PH.D.

At this writing, Colin Campbell, Ph.D., is the Jacob Gould Schurman Professor Emeritus of Nutritional Biochemistry at Cornell University in Ithaca, New York. He has authored over 300 scientific papers and served as Senior Science Adviser to the American Institute for Cancer Research/World Research Fund.

As Director of the China-Oxford-Cornell Study, one of the biggest,

ADDING DAIRY *BLOCKS* TEA'S CARDIOVASCULAR BENEFITS

German researchers out of Germany found that drinking tea can reduce the risk of heart disease and stroke, but *only if milk is not added* to the beverage.

Tea has been shown to improve blood flow and the arteries ability to relax. However, adding milk eliminates tea's protective effect against cardiovascular disease. "If you want to drink tea to have the beneficial health effects you have to drink it without milk. That is clearly shown by our experiments," said Dr. Verena Stangl, a cardiologist at the Hospital at the University of Berlin (MSNBC 2007).

Stangl and her researchers found that proteins called caseins in milk actually decrease the amount of catechins in tea, which help to protect against heart disease. Tea has also been shown to have a protective effect against cancer, so the findings from this study may have further implications.

most comprehensive studies of disease and diet ever mounted, Dr. Campbell and colleagues measured 367 diet, lifestyle, and disease-related variables in 65 counties in rural China and Taiwan. The study involved 6500 adults aged 35 to 64 who filled out diet questionnaires, had blood and urine tests, and had their food purchases analyzed.

Why China? Because in China, there is huge variation between geographic areas in the incidence of diseases such as cancer. This intrigued Dr. Campbell and his colleagues at Oxford University in England. In people who didn't differ by much genetically—all the subjects were of the same race—a special opportunity presented itself to study the influence of diet on disease risk.

At the outset, it was obvious that the Chinese consume far more iron, plant foods, fiber, and calories per kilogram of body weight than Americans. They also consume far less fat, total protein, and animal protein. The Chinese subjects have a 20 percent lower average body mass index than Americans—in other words, they are slimmer despite eating more calories than we do, even those Chinese who were not physically active.

The results? That the cause of degenerative diseases—not just bone loss, but also cardiovascular disease and cancer—is a diet too high in animal protein and lacking in nutrient-dense plant foods (vegetables, fruit, legumes). Not surprisingly, Dr. Campbell's work is often referred to by those who would like to promote the causes of vegetarianism and veganism, and by those who wish to ditch the dairy calcium standard so prevalent in developed nations today.

Dr. Campbell grew up on a dairy farm. As a child, he milked cows and guzzled huge amounts of fresh milk every day, and ate lots of meat. But in the course of becoming a respected scientist and college professor, and in the course of mounting the China Study, he swore off dairy and meat for life, and doesn't give it to his children or grandchildren.

MILK AND CROHN'S DISEASE: IS THERE A LINK?

Crohn's disease is an intestinal disorder that is akin to the worst stomach flu you've ever had—only it flares up repeatedly and may be constant throughout the rest of your life. Usually, it develops during the teen years or the early 20s. The rate of Crohn's disease cases has risen sharply since the 1940s, and is now at the highest rate ever recorded.

Crohn's disease is a form of *inflammatory bowel disease* (IBD), a class of diseases that also includes a less severe form called *ulcerative colitis*. In people with this disease, the lining of the small and/or large intestine becomes extremely inflamed. It can develop ulcers or even *fistulas*, where inflammation spreads out to other organs or even out of the body through the skin.

About half a million Americans suffer from some form of IBD. Those who are diagnosed with Crohn's or ulcerative colitis are told that their disease is incurable; that they can expect to cycle through periods of flare-up and remission; and that they will likely require intense drug therapy, which often causes serious side effects, to control the disease.

Medical authorities claim that no one knows what causes it, although they do know that it tends to run in families and that diet changes can help reduce flare-ups. As is so often the case, however, modern medicine understates the potential role of dietary triggers in the genesis of this devastating condition. An overloaded liver and gallbladder has been associated with this malady. (see references on seasonal cleanses for symptoms)

What could be a plausible dietary cause? Some authorities have made compelling arguments supporting a link between Crohn's disease (as well as *irritable bowel syndrome,* a more minor digestive problem that usually involves some combination of gas, flatulence, diarrhea, and constipation) and a type of bacteria that commonly appears in cow's milk. That bacterium is called *mycobacterium paratuberculosis* (MAP), and it is found in the milk of cows infected with Johne's disease—the bovine version of Crohn's.

According to a study published in 1965, 100 percent of people with Crohn's disease test positive for the paratuberculosis bacteria. It is not eliminated during the milk pasteurization process.

Coincidentally, the dairy industry is seeing a rise in Johne's disease among cattle. Clinical epidemiological and DNA evidence points to MAP as the cause of Crohn's disease in humans. The MAP bacteria is found within pus cells, which are found in higher concentrations in American dairy milk than any other country—up to twice as much as the allowable international standard of allowable pus levels. That's right: when you down that cool, creamy glass of milk, you're drinking pus.

In one study performed in Sardinia, Italy, college students with Crohn's disease and IBS had intestinal biopsies for MAP, as did a group of healthy control subjects. Local dairy sheep were also tested for the bug. The results were compelling: the bacterium was detected in samples from 15 of 20 patients with IBS; 20 of 23 patients with Crohn's disease; and 3 of 20 control subjects. Seven of eight dairy sheep tested positive for MAP, and the likelihood of having Crohn's or IBS was greater in those who reported having eaten local sheep's-milk cheese.

Johne's disease is a serious problem in U.S. dairy cattle. It afflicts three quarters of a million cattle—20 to 40 percent of dairy herds. Some suggest that cattle overcrowding is the culprit. More and more cattle are left to graze on smaller plots of land, forcing the cows to live, eat, and excrete in close proximity, which would, naturally, contribute to bacterial growth and spread.

Although the dairy industry would like us to believe that MAP is eliminated in the pasteurization process, researchers in Ireland have proved otherwise. In 1998, Irish researchers grew live paratuberculosis bacteria out of 6 of the 31 cartons of pasteurized milk they tested—that's 20 percent, or 1 in 5! While this caused a media stir across Europe, where the epidemic was called "enormous" and "horrific," not a headline was made here in the U.S. Not surprising, considering the damage that would certainly be done to the dairy industry if this news got out stateside.

Studies conducted by Rorick Chiodini, a microbiologist at Brown University's Rhode Island Hospital, definitively showed the presence of paraturberculosis bacteria in the gut walls of children with Crohn's disease. Chiodini wrote, "the dairy and regulatory industries are concerned vocally . . . but their concern is limited to the possibility of 'bad press' to the industry *rather than a concern for the truth or public health."*

Why is it that countries such as Ireland exclude cattle infected with Johne's disease for human consumption, but the U.S. does not? Ireland strictly forbids humans from eating diseased flesh or drinking milk from an infected cow, yet here at home we are consuming meat and milk that is tainted with paratuberculosis. Dr. John Hermon-Taylor, chairman of the surgery department at St. George's Medical School in London and an internationally known expert on Crohn's and paratuberculosis, has said of this issue that "[t]here is overwhelming evidence that we are sitting on a public health disaster of tragic proportions."

Perhaps if we were to heed these warnings from these international experts we would see a decrease in the escalating number of people suffering from Crohn's disease. At this point, every few hours a child is diagnosed with Crohn's and is sentenced to a lifetime of suffering. It's time to stop the madness!

LACTOSE INTOLERANCE IS EXTREMELY COMMON

Caucasians are most likely to have the ability through childhood and adulthood to make the enzyme *lactase,* which breaks down lactose—milk sugar—in the digestive tract. People of Asian and African descent are significantly likely to lack this enzyme, which means diarrhea, gas, bloating, and pain when dairy products are consumed.

Health authorities have claimed that even lactose intolerant people can, with practice, get to the point where small amounts of dairy can be eaten. To *not* encourage this practice, they say, is "racist"—how could we deprive these other races of the vast health benefits of dairy foods?

If you've gotten this far in this book, you know how ridiculous this is. Most of the world's people do just fine without the so-called "health benefits" of dairy. The longest-lived, healthiest people on earth are those who consume calcium in the form of vegetables, fruit, and legumes, and consume little or no dairy. (The China Study–Cormnell–Oxford University)

Who's really racist here—those who want to tell the truth about the risks of dairy and to recommend far healthier alternatives, or those who would subject people whose bodies wisely reject dairy foods to repeated bouts of painful gas, flatulence, and diarrhea?

AMERICAN rBGH MILK BANNED IN EUROPE, CANADA, AUSTRALIA, NEW ZEALAND & JAPAN!

We milk-guzzling Americans expect a lot from our cows. We expect to be able to get our three a day of dairy without having it be expensive. So we developed technology that made cows produce more milk, faster. As often happens when we fool with mother Nature, this practice seems to have come around to bite us.

In November 1993, the Food and Drug Administration (FDA) approved the injection of American dairy cows with genetically-engineered bovine growth hormone (rBGH) to increase milk production. This practice works, no question: with rBGH injections, cows produce up to 20 times more milk.

Unfortunately, this growth hormone also stimulates the cows' livers to increase levels of *insulin-like growth factor* (IGF-1) in their milk. This modified, IGF-

---

GOT . . . MUCUS?

If you're health-conscious, you have likely heard somewhere that dairy consumption can worsen congestion. Is this an urban legend . . . or is there some scientific foundation to the idea that milk does mucus good?

Mucus is formed by the immune system in response to an irritant or allergen. The offending substance stimulates the production of *histamine*, a chemical formed by the immune system that Its job is to sweep up the irritating substance and get it out of the body through coughing, sneezing, or a runny nose. Mucus can sometimes form in the intestinal tract as the body tries to remove irritants from the bowel.

Milk contains proteins that are irritating or allergenic to many people. When dairy products are consumed, these proteins end up in the bloodstream, activating histamine production and leading to increased mucus production. Eliminating dairy often helps those with chronic congestion; sometimes, they find complete relief with this one small change.

---

impregnated milk is known to increase the risk of breast, colon and prostate cancers. Once a human consumes rBGH milk, IGF-1 is not destroyed by the human digestive system. Instead, IGF-1 is easily and readily absorbed across the intestinal wall and bloodstream, where it impacts other hormones. The same goes for other hormones and bioactive compounds found in cow's milk, including estrogens.

Once consumed, IGF-1 encourages the transformation of normal breast cells to breast cancers. Also, IGF-1 maintains the malignancy of human breast cancer cells, boosting their ability to spread and invade other organs such as the prostate and colon.

The hazards of this IGF-1 infusion are so real that European nations and Canada have *banned* American milk containing rBGH. But in the U.S., the FDA has been downright hostile in response to critics who suggest that milk containing rBGH should indicate so on the labels. This, they claim, would somehow imply that the non-rBGH milk is better than the rBGH milk, and well, we just don't know that to be true . . . yet.

Of course, this is a government that failed to protect citizens against asbestos, leaded gasoline, mercury in vaccines, methylmercury and other toxic chemical contaminants in the foods we eat, and various other very nasty drugs and chemicals . . . until the evidence was so overwhelming that many people had already been injured or killed.

Here's some of what we do know about rBGH: In 1990, the National Institutes of Health Consensus panel on rBGH expressed serious concerns about the adverse health effects of IGF-1 in rBGH milk, calling for further studies on how it impacts health, particularly for infants. In 1991, the Council on Scientific Affairs of the American Medical Association stated, "Further studies will be required to determine whether the ingestion of higher than normal concentrations of bovine insulin-like growth factor is safe for children, adolescents and adults." But . . . *these studies were never done!* Cows injected with rBGH have heavy localization of IGF-1 in their udder (breast) epithelial cells, which is not the case in cows not injected with rBGH. rBGH-injected cows have an 80 percent increased risk of udder infections, or mastitis. Through their infected udders, milk becomes contaminated by significant levels of white blood cells, also known as somatic cells or pus, which must be treated by antibiotics. The residue of the pus and the antibiotics are passed from the udders through the milk for human consumption. And these are not minute amounts of pus: one to seven drops of these cells are in every eight-ounce glass of milk! This can vary by state to state, but only *one* state out of all fifty has a cell count lower than the dairy industry's recommendations. And seventeen states within the U.S. produce milk that would be *illegal* to sell based on somatic cell limits in Europe. The evidence linking IGF-1 and cancer is mounting. The European Commission released a report by its 16 member scientific committee that confirmed excess levels of IGF-1 in cow milk to the rise in breast and prostate cancer incidences. According to the Cancer Prevention Coalition's 2003 report, "[e]xperimental evidence for an association between IGF-1 and breast and prostate cancer is supported by epidemiological evidence arising from recently published cohort studies." The report goes on to warn that excess levels of IGF-1 may encourage the growth and invasiveness of any cancer by inhibiting programmed self-destruction of cancer cells. This same report points out that contamination of milk with residues of antibiotics used to treat udder infections in cows is likely to spread antibiotic-resistant infections in humans.

The European Commission's report is in stark contrast to those who are responsible for setting American food safety standards. Those authorities gave an unqualified clean bill of health to rBGH milk!

The public is getting wise on this front, and due to pressure from consumers, American retailers appear to be getting smarter. On June 9, 2006, the largest milk processor in the world and the two largest supermarkets in the United States (Dean Foods, Wal-Mart and Kroger) announced that they are on a nationwide search for rBGH-free milk.

In January of 2007, Starbucks Corporation announced that it is banning rBGH-infused milk and other dairy products from its stores throughout the United States. This move came after Starbucks was singled out in a campaign by consumer groups who are avidly against the use of rBGH milk.

Starbucks spokesman Brandon Borman was quoted as saying, "We are actively engaged with all our dairy suppliers to explore converting our core dairy products to be rBGH-free in our U.S. company-owned stores. This is something that our customers have requested." (CNN 2007).

This is *exactly* what we consumers need to do to demand the needed changes that protect our health and that of our loved ones. Clearly, because rBGH is not allowed in other countries, Starbucks only has to make the changes here in the U.S. Finally, we're catching on to what the rest of the world already knows.

Until labels are updated, unless the milk label states "No rBGH," you can assume that the milk you drink is contaminated with a chemical, biological and bacterial cocktail.

MILK AND CANCER: INCREASING EVIDENCE OF A CAUSAL LINK

Nations that consume the most dairy are not only at highest risk of osteoporosis; they are also at highest risk of cancer. Coincidence? Probably not. Although dairy is not the only potential cause of cancer in developed nations—far from it!—it's naïve to think, based on current research, that it is not a contributing factor.

Truth be told, milk is chock-full of hormones, including estrogens, progesterone, insulin, and naturally occurring growth hormones, along with other bioactive substances. Cow's milk is a specialized natural soup, designed through millions of years of evolution, to promote growth in baby cows, just as human milk is a specialized natural soup designed to promote growth in baby humans. Adding extra growth hormones is adding insult to injury, but there is a reason you don't want to pour human breastmilk on your cereal—because somewhere in the depths of your consciousness, you understand that milk is not an appropriate food for adults. Cow's milk is culturally sanctioned in the U.S. and seems like a normal food, and so we move past this natural distaste—but should we? The majority of the evidence seems to shout, "No!"

And let's not disregard the fact that fat-soluble, carcinogenic industrial toxins, including dioxins, concentrate in fatty foods like milk. Cutting down on animal-derived foods like meat and dairy will cut down on your body's continual accumulation of these toxins, which may help to protect against cancer.

Estrogens in cow's milk are particularly worrisome with regard to heightened cancer risk. In the bodies of mammals, estrogen's job is to promote increased cell growth. This means that estrogen not only encourages the growth of bone cells—it also has this effect on cancer cells. This is why it helps prevent bone loss when given as a drug; and this is why it is listed in medical and toxicology texts as a known carcinogen. Especially vulnerable to the effects of excess estrogen: the tissues of the breasts and prostate gland.

A study by the Department of Nutrition, Harvard School of Public Health in Boston did research for 11 years looking at a high calcium intake, mainly from dairy products, and its impact on the risk of prostate cancer. Out of 20,885 men, the researchers documents 1,012 cases of prostate cancer. The researchers found that compared to men consuming under 150 mg of calcium from dairy products, men who consumed 600mg a day of dairy had a 32 percent *higher risk* of prostate cancer (Chan 2001).

Hungarian researchers analyzed the risk of breast cancer with respect to IGF-1, IGF-binding globulin-3 and testosterone to predict hormone-dependent breast cancer in post-menopausal women. They concluded that there was an increased prevalence of breast cancers in patients with higher levels of IGF-1, IGFBP-3 or testosterone (Kahan 2006). Despite these and other indicative findings, the FDA has failed to further investigate the long-term effects of IGF-1 and treated milk on growth.

MILK HELPS YOU LOSE WEIGHT: FACT OR FICTION?

More advertising genius on the part of the dairy industry: the ads that show a svelte startlet with a milk mustache who tells us that her three-a-day milk habit helps her stay slim. Studies have shown that a weight-loss diet—consisting of fewer calories taken in than calories burned—can be "amped up" with three glasses of milk a day. These studies have given dairy producers the right to plaster their products with slogans like "Lose More Weight!" and "Burn More Fat!" to encourage sales.

This claim is based on research by University of Tennessee professor Michael Zemel, who found that this much milk accelerated weight loss in a group of dieters. All of his subjects went on a reduced-calorie diet; some drank the USDA's recommended amount of milk and some drank no milk, and the milk drinkers lost almost twice as much weight.

Balance this weight-loss excitement with the fact that simply adding dairy to your current diet will NOT help you lose weight—in fact, you'll most likely gain from the extra calories. Dr. Zemel has made this point clear. Also consider that most studies on this subject find no connection between weight loss and dairy product consumption, and that some demonstrate that those who consume more dairy actually stand at higher risk of *gaining* weight.

I'd like to see a comparison between Dr. Zemel's weight-loss diet with three-a-day dairy and the same diet with three-a-day servings of calcium-rich vegetables and legumes. I think I know who'd win *that* head-to-head.

DAIRY AND ACNE: THE HORMONE LINK

Do you know a teen or young adult who suffers from acne? Zits are a big problem for young people, and modern medicine tends to treat it with medications both topical and systemic. Millions upon millions of dollars are spent each year on cosmetic products touted as anti-acne agents, and more yet on cosmetics designed to mask blemishes. But the link between diet—which, in the case of most teens, is truly lacking in just about everything healthful and chock-full of sugar, refined carbohydrates, bad fats, and dairy—and acne is swept under the rug by most medical authorities.

Everyone knows that adolescent acne is about the surge of hormones that is changing that child to an adult. When a cow is milked during its pregnancy and that milk is consumed by that teen, a soup of hormones is added to the already potent mix coursing through his or her body. This milk contains *androgens* like testosterone, and these androgens directly affect sebaceous (oil) glands in the skin and can promote acne.

Another culprit: refined sugars and flour—foods that cause insulin levels to spike, and over time, to remain elevated. High levels of insulin promote sebum production in sebaceous glands, setting the stage for the acne explosion.

The dairy-acne link is supported by research from the Harvard School of Public Health. In one study of 4,273 teen boys, food frequency questionnaires were given, and they reported their history of acne. Boys who consumed the most dairy (more than two servings a day) had significantly higher incidence of self-reported acne than those who consumed the least (less than one serving per week). Another study of 6,094 teen girls found an even stronger link than the study of teen boys.

In conclusion, the researchers wrote, "We found a positive association with acne for intake of total milk and skim milk. We hypothesize that the association with milk may be because of the presence of hormones and bioactive molecules in milk."

How many teens do you know who regard sugary cereal with milk as a staple of their diet? Personally, I've known quite a few. If you know someone who's tormented by zits that won't go away, you may want to propose that he or she give up dairy, refined sugars, and foods made from flour.

MILK AND TYPE 1 DIABETES

Childhood-onset diabetes is on the rise in Western countries. In this disease, which differs substantially from the adult-onset, type 2 diabetes described on pages 61–62, the pancreas—a gland located along the small intestine—becomes unable to make insulin. Insulin's job is to move glucose, the simplest form of carbohydrate, out of the bloodstream and into the cells so that it can be burned as energy. When a child's body loses the ability to produce enough insulin, he or she requires insulin injections for survival. Even with good blood sugar control, a child with type 1 diabetes faces a much-heightened lifetime risk of heart disease, kidney failure, blinding eye disease, and nerve damage—not to mention a daily risk of falling into insulin shock or diabetic coma if anything goes wrong with his or her medication schedule.

What is the cause of this terrifying disease? A vitamin D deficiency has been associated with this challenge. One controversial but compelling theory: a mismatch between the child's immune system and the proteins found in milk. It appears that the immune systems of some children react so strongly to milk proteins that the insulin-producing cells in the pancreas are destroyed. Another compelling theory: that a young child or baby's immune system recognizes that the cow insulin found in cow's milk—which differs from human insulin, but only very slightly—and attacks it. By association, the immune systems of some children may end up attacking their body's own insulin-making cells.

Longer duration of breastfeeding (including six months of exclusive breastfeeding, with no other food or beverages) and delaying introduction of cow's milk are both known to reduce risk of type 1 diabetes. Don't buy the party line that your child needs to guzzle cow's milk to be healthy. As good as vegetable, nut, and legume sources of calcium are for adults, they are even better for children, once they are ready for solid food.

Milk Isn't the Answer For Strong Bones

This may have been a tough chapter for you. Dairy foods are tasty and comforting. It can be hard to imagine a life without cheese, cream, milk, ice cream, and yogurt.

I am not saying that dairy-free is the only way to live. My point here is that milk and other dairy foods aren't going to protect your bones, and if you over consume them they may cause or promote digestive problems, congestion, weight gain, acne, or even breast or prostate cancer. If you love dairy foods and want to enjoy them in small amounts, and you don't perceive that your body reacts to them in any untoward fashion, enjoy them every so often. Personally, I love to have the occasional bit of organic, hormone free cheese or ice cream!—but I don't rely on them to fill any of my nutritional requirements.

American nutritionists and the USDA are giving people a false sense of security with its calcium/dairy guidelines. They give the impression that our best hope of achieving calcium adequacy is with our three a day of dairy. But, as you've seen in this chapter, the calcium in milk has not been found to promote or preserve bone health. And it quite possibly may be *damaging your* bones.

In this book, I'll give you all the information and recipes you need to get adequate bone-building nutrition *without dairy products*. In the meantime: don't rely on dairy products to give you adequate calcium. And if you have chronic health problems or concerns, and you never considered that dairy products might be a cause, you may want to start considering that those cheesy, creamy dairy delights might be at the root of it.

Chapter Four

Osteoporosis:
IT'S NOT JUST FOR THE ELDERLY

One of the most life-shattering events that can happen to any person is a broken hip. In the U.S., bone fractures have become a 21st century plague. Death rates from falls have risen dramatically since the 1990s.

When bones are weak to begin with, only the smallest tumble is required to shatter a hip. Tumbling from a ladder or down a flight of stairs isn't necessary to have this end result. Weak, brittle bones in the spine, hips, and wrists can snap like twigs during the performance of menial, everyday tasks. Even bending over, sneezing, carrying groceries, or tripping over a curb can be the instigating event in a person with fragile bones.

According to the U.S. Surgeon General, hip fractures are the most devastating type of bone fracture, putting more than 300,000 people in the hospital each year. An estimated 20 percent of hospitalized individuals with hip fractures will die within a year of their hospitalization, while another 20 percent will end up "warehoused" in a nursing home. Sadly, the vast majority of others who suffer a hip fracture must cope with severe physical limitations. Losing one's mobility often leads to isolation and helplessness, which then leads to feelings of depression.

The Surgeon General warns that approximately 10 million Americans over the age of 50 have osteoporosis, and that 34 million more are at risk. Most of these people, however, don't know their bones are becoming increasingly fragile. There are no "red flag" signs to set off the alarm bells. The only way to know that bones are deteriorating, short of a catastrophic, painful fracture, is to have a bone mineral density test. And all too often, the problem is only detected in this way when it's already advanced and risk of fracture is high.

If these trends aren't reversed, at least half of all Americans over 50 will have weakened bones from osteoporosis by the year 2020. One in two baby-boomer women is projected to sustain an osteoporotic bone fracture after the age of 50. That's a staggering implication: *one in two* Americans at risk for bone fractures from osteoporosis or low bone mass! Popping the usual calcium supplements doesn't look like a promising solution. With whole food calcium supplements and the Whole Body Bone Building diet and lifestyle, however, I'm confident that this picture could become considerably more hopeful.

SYMPTOMS OF OSTEOPOROSIS

In its early stages, osteoporosis doesn't usually have symptoms. Once advanced, it may be felt as dull pain in the back (especially the lumbar spine, or low back) and neck. Further along, the person with osteoporosis is likely to experience sharp, sudden pains that may or may not radiate. The pain can get worse if weight is put on the area, and tends to start to subside after about a week but can linger for three months or more. Very advanced disease can cause a substantial loss of height, or a dowager's hump, where the upper back curves forward.

OSTEOPOROSIS IS A MAN'S DISEASE, TOO— AND A DISEASE OF THE YOUNG

Contrary to popular belief, weakened bones are *not* just a woman's problem, nor a natural result of aging. If any person—man, woman, or child—is not fulfilling bone-nourishing requirements, they are left vulnerable to bone fractures that can be challenging at any stage of life. While we hear a lot of news reports warning that women must get their daily calcium to prevent osteoporosis, there is an *underreporting* of what may be required by men and children.

Approximately one-third of bone weight is made up of a protein matrix rich in a variety of minerals, nutrients, and amino acids, including magnesium, sodium, copper, potassium, zinc, manganese,vitamin B3, lysine, silica, vitamin C, vitamin D, chromium, folic acid, boron, essential fatty acids, vitamin A, selenium, phytosterols, and calcium. Good lifestyle habits combined with all of these substances play a crucial role in providing the elements needed to achieve strong, healthy bones.

At every age and stage of life, human bone constantly undergoes changes. In fact, some bones in our bodies are *completely regenerated* every three months. This breaking down and building of bone is a natural and necessary process that enables the skeleton to naturally strengthen and heal itself.

Think of a home remodeling project. As one wall is knocked down, a new adjacent wall goes up. To prevent structural damage, it is important to maintain a fine balance between building and destruction; otherwise, you might find your home has collapsed into a pile of rubble. And this is true of the bone remodeling process, too—for every age and sex.

As bone cells, called osteoblasts, continuously create new bone, other bone cells called osteoclasts are busy breaking down and removing old, tired bone. This remodeling process takes place throughout life, but the building aspect slows as we age. The older we get, the less bone our bodies build to replace what's broken down . . . *unless* we continually stimulate new bone growth with stellar nutrition and weight-bearing exercise. Use it or lose it! Feed it or waste it! You have more control than you probably know. With your choices, you can make a huge difference in your own bone health.

Because children and men have been neglected by the public health push for better bone mass, I'm hoping that the women who read this will use what they've learned to help their children and spouses. It's never too soon, or too late, to start.

THE TRUTH ABOUT WOMEN'S RISK FACTORS

It is true that women over the age of 50 have the greatest risk of developing osteoporosis. Because of lighter, thinner bones combined with a long life-span, women tend to be at a higher risk for osteoporosis than men.

While the common perception is that osteoporosis is a "white woman's disease," the reality is that Asian and African-American women also face a significant risk of developing osteoporosis—when they live in a Western country, embrace a sedentary Western lifestyle, and eat a Western diet.

Bone structure and body weight also play a role when determining risk factors. For example, small-boned, petite, thin women (under 127 pounds) have a greater risk of developing osteoporosis because they have less bone to lose than women with larger frames. Slighter-framed men also have heightened risk of osteoporotic changes.

Menopause plays a role in bone loss in women—but not as big a role as you might believe based on what you've been told by your doctor. Estrogen helps to slow down the rate of bone loss by inhibiting the activity of osteoblast cells whose job it is to break down bone. Estrogen production falls at menopause for some women, and at that point, bone loss can accelerate. World-renowned calcium and osteoporosis researcher Robert Heaney, PhD, and others have found that both low calcium intake *and* menopause are overrated in their role in causing osteoporosis.

One reason why this menopause-osteoporosis connection has been so played up: to sell pharmaceuticals. If estrogen lack is the key to bone loss, then estrogen replacement would seem to be the best solution; and for decades, estrogen replacement drugs like Premarin were top sellers worldwide as osteoporosis preventives.

Bone protection is one of the key reasons why many women once opted for hormone replacement therapy (HRT). Since research revealed unacceptable increases in risk of heart problems and breast cancer with long-term use of HRT, the many millions of women who once relied on this therapy to keep their bones strong are seeking other alternatives. The study was alarming enough for the federal government to add *all* estrogens to their updated list of 228 known carcinogens (cancer-causing substances) in 2002.

Women's bodies continue to make some estrogen following

menopause. It's made in fat cells and by the adrenals; it follows that women who are heavier are less likely to need extra estrogen. Women can also consume plant estrogens—phytosterols from herbs like dong quai, suma, ginseng, wild yam, black cohosh, dandelion, red clover, yarrow, sage, and fenugreek, and from foods like tofu and miso—to naturally protect bone with gentle, balanced, whole-food estrogenic stimulation. (More on soy isoflavones shortly.)

MENOPAUSE DOESN'T HAVE TO MEAN WEAK BONES

Women who eat calcium-rich foods and exercise regularly through-out their adult lives enter their menopausal years with better bone mass than women who are sedentary and consume calcium-leaching foods (including coffee, sodas, alcohol, salt, dairy, chocolate, and processed meats). They have more bone mass to start with, and so they have more to spare if bone loss does accelerate a bit at menopause.

Minerals complexed naturally in green plants seem to be ideal for keeping bones healthy. "The closer people get to a diet based on plant foods and leafy vegetables, the lower the rates of many diseases, including osteoporosis," says Dr. Colin Campbell, whose research you learned about in Chapter 3. In his China-Oxford-Cornell Study, women in rural China with the lowest known fracture rates were those who ate the most calcium-rich plants and who exercised regularly. These women lowered their risk of osteoporosis exponentially. This is huge! We must learn from these study's as they are the key's to our happier, healthier lives.

With the onset of menopause, there can be a brief period of "bone-pause," occurring off and on for five to seven years—after which things calm down and bone loss slows again. Whole food calcium supplements with all the complementary nutrients I recommend in this book, plus plenty of calcium-rich vegetables and exercise, can make all the difference during these years and those that follow.

Unfortunately, most women aren't hip to this advice quite yet, and by the age of 40, many American women are well on their way to losing serious bone mass; by the age of 50, hormones or drugs are often prescribed to try to slow this process down. With the dangers of standard HRT better known than ever before, women are taking on inappropriate risks by using these drugs for even this length of time.

The five to seven year "bone-pause" period does pass, after which time the bones *can* rebuild themselves—especially when supported by nourishing herbs and other plant calcium sources, which are exceptional sources of bone-building minerals and cofactors and better at preventing bone breaks than standard calcium salts (carbonate, gluconate, citrate, phosphates, and coral calcium). This is an important time to make sure calcium and calcium cofactor intake is generous, and that the form of calcium used is easily assimilated, utilized, and retained by the body.

To Soy or Not To Soy? The Isoflavone Conundrum

Research unequivocally shows that soyfoods rich in isoflavones (the plant's phytosterols, which are weakly estrogenic) helps to build bone. But the agreement on soy isoflavones seems to end there.

Some tout soyfoods as great allies to one's health; others demonize them as nutritional no-nos. Some research seems to suggest that soy isoflavones are beneficial to women's health, protecting against female cancers and heart disease, while other studies indicate that soy isoflavones could actually *increase* breast cancer risk. And although calcium-processed tofu is billed as a good calcium source, soy is a very common food allergen , full of antinutrients that can disrupt absorption of minerals and may even impede thyroid function. (This occurs because most soy on the market is isolated in America and has had many of its most important (phytoestrogens, vitamin E, phytosterols, saponins, selenium, potassium, isoflavones, genistein, diadzene, plant protein, . . .) nutrient constituents altered or stripped.)

So: the next time you find yourself standing in front of a shelf full of soyfoods in the supermarket, or in front of a shelf containing supplement bottles full of isoflavone pills or jars of isoflavone-enriched soy protein, what should you do? Here are a few pointers that will help you decide which, if any, to take home and feed to yourself and your family.

- Traditionally prepared, non-isolated or unprocessed soyfoods, eaten in moderation, are good for your bones, heart, and body. One to two servings per day of calcium-prepared tofu, edamame (green soybeans in their pods), miso (fermented soybean paste), or tempeh (fermented soybeans formed into a block that can be prepared much as one might prepare meat) will give you all the isoflavones you need—up to 100 mg of soy isoflavones per day. Some is good; more is not better!

- Soy expert Mark Messina, Ph.D., of Loma Linda University in southern California, suggests that women with a history of breast cancer only consume two to three servings of (unprocessed) soyfoods per week. The same recommendation would be wisely followed by a woman who knows that breast cancer runs in her family. It's important to understand as much as possible how the right kind of soy works for our health. The two isoflavones-genistein & diadzein-act like weak estrogens in the body-in a good way though. These isoflavones compete with stronger naturally occurring estrogens to help prevent hormone dependent cancers such as prostate and breast. The isoflavones bind to sites on cell membranes that normally would be inhabited by hormones that stimulate these cancers. Thus they block the action of the strong hormones as well as they inhibit the enzyme activity that would otherwise stimulate the growth of tumors and blood clots. Once again, the truth is that when we consume the isolated, processed forms of this plant it becomes deleterious to our health.

- Soymilk is high in isoflavones. All that I have seen are processed and have isolated calcium and other synthetic nutrients in them. You can make your own with frozen or fresh soybeans in water blended into a frothy milk with out the sugars and additives. You can make your own other non-dairy milks: almond, rice, and hemp milks and are all nice additions to a plant-based diet.

- As I said before, the same whole-food principles that should guide calcium supplementation also guide isoflavone intake. Avoid taking supplements that contain isolated, concentrated soy isoflavones. The jury isn't even close to in on what the effects of these supplements might be, or whether they could increase risk of breast cancer. They have been stripped of their cofactors that guide the important nutrients in the bean to where they could have been must beneficial.
- The same goes for concentrated soy protein, which is a common ingredient in protein powders, nutrition bars, and processed foods you may find in the "healthy" section of your supermarket.

THE STARTLING TRUTH ABOUT CHILDREN'S BONE HEALTH

In recent years, emergency rooms and doctors' offices have seen an astounding rise in the number of children with broken bones. According to a 2004 study of orthopedic surgeons and pediatricians, more than 40 percent of doctors have observed a surge in fractures in people under the age of 18. Two other medical studies found that the rate of broken arms has jumped by more than 50 percent in girls and 30 percent in boys since the 1970s. This includes a 33 percent increase in forearm breaks.

Most amazing is the *kind* of break being seen in children. The bone breaks like chalk—it crumbles. This seems to be a direct reflection of the use of calcium from chalk as fortification in the foods and supplements women consume while pregnant, and in the foods routinely fed to children—foods and supplements that also do not contain the needed minerals and cofactors. This calcium can't interconnect properly to make the solid but flexible bone matrix that naturally occurs in young children.

Ceila Brown, M.D., puts it this way: "What used to be bruises are more likely to be breaks nowadays . . . Kids just aren't developing adequate bone mass." (Got Milk 2001).

From birth until around the age of 18, bones are forming and growing. Calcium, vitamin D, and at least 17 other nutrient with their cofactors are *essential* to this critical process. Babies get enough calcium from breast milk and infant formulas, but as children grow, they need to maintain a calcium-rich diet to ensure strong bones.

Unfortunately, the calcium intake of most American children peaks at eight years old. Preschoolers have the benefit of their parents choosing their diet, but after around the age of eight, these kids tend to make most of their own decisions. And any parent knows what those decisions tend to be: pasteurized, sugary juice or soda instead of water or fresh-squeezed juices or superfood antioxidant drinks; unhealthy snacks such as chips or cookies over calcium-rich veggies and legumes; and anything with sugar in it rules over virtually anything else.

Through late adolescence and young adulthood, adult bones are forming and reach their maximum strength and density, but still require additional calcium long after these growth spurts have come and gone. The calcium you feed your bones when you are young determines how well they will hold up throughout their lifetime.

While bone weakness usually doesn't manifest as osteoporosis until one is getting well on in years, getting off to a good start in early childhood is the best preventative measure a person can take. Throughout one's lifetime, old bone is removed from the skeleton and new bone is created. During childhood and the teen years, new bone is added faster than old bone is removed, making a positive bone balance. The result is larger, heavier, denser bones that are better prepared to fight off bone loss with age.

The serious rise in broken bones is partly due to a lack of appropriate calcium, vitamin D, approximately 17 other vital minerals and nutrients during their childhood and teen years. Government studies indicate that 86 percent of teen girls and 64 percent of teen boys are not getting enough usable or retainable calcium daily. These are frightening numbers. If this trend continues unchecked, these children will be faced with a lifetime of bone-related challenges that will not only limit their abilities, negatively influence their lifestyle and possibly shorten their life span. The USDA estimates that only

37 to 40 percent of kids aged two to 17 are getting the daily recommended amounts of calcium.

Add to this worrisome news: young women who take oral contraceptives (birth control pills) and get regular exercise have actually been found to *lose* bone mass—right at the time of life where building all the bone one can is key. In one study, women on the Pill and women not on the Pill were put on similarly intense workout programs, and the women not on the Pill made significant gains in bone density, while those popping the oral contraceptives gained no bone density at all. Why? Most likely due to the effects of synthetic progestins, which are drugs found in all birth control pills. Progestins are similar to human progesterone, but actually "block" the effects of the real thing. And one of progesterone's important effects on a woman's body is to build bone.

Young women with eating disorders are at special risk of osteoporosis. A study of 130 young women with anorexia nervosa found that half had spinal and hip osteopenia (a sort of pre-osteoporosis, where bone loss is already significant) and between 13 and 24 percent had outright osteoporosis in these areas.

Habitual "yo-yo" dieters—those who go to calorie-cutting and workout extremes to lose weight fast, then regain it and end up working even harder to lose it again—are also at risk. People who work out regularly to lose weight or achieve fitness or athletic goals need two to three times more nourishment than couch potatoes, which makes the right supplements even more necessary for them.

Even children who are taking in adequate amounts of bone-fortifying nutrients remain at risk of losing bone density. Typical kids' diets contain bone-leaching foods and drinks. One of the biggest calcium-leaching offenders is soft drinks—especially caffeine-rich sodas. Colas contain phosphates, which are known calcium thieves. An analysis of about 1,400 elderly participants in the Framingham study found that the more caffeinated colas participants consumed, the lower their bone density was likely to be. Our kids, today, are starting to guzzle these beverages from a young age, and their bones are likely to suffer over time.

A 2004 study of broken bones found that substituting sodas for milk could be an important cause. In fact, forty two percent of the doctors cited low milk consumption and inadequate calcium intake for the skyrocketing rise in broken bones in kids. (See Chapter 3 for the real truth about dairy).

Worried? You should be, according to Leon Root, MD and author of *Beautiful Bones Without Hormones* and professor of clinical orthopedics at Weill Medical College of Cornell University in New York City. "Osteoporosis is actually a childhood disease that manifests itself later in life," he explains.

Nothing, but nothing, makes me cringe more than to hear a two- or three- year-old asking their parents for a soda—except, perhaps, to hear the child's parent agreeing to hand one over! Young children need calcium-*building* foods and drinks to make sure their bones get a strong start. These calcium-leaching dietary habits are definitely not setting the stage for a strong skeletal foundation.

Soda and other caffeinated drinks, such as coffee or tea, are literally *robbing* children and adults alike of the calcium they get from food. Nutrition surveys have found that young kids are drinking nearly 15 ounces of soda per day, and that teens are drinking anywhere from 20 to 30 ounces of soda a day. Removing sodas from schools is a good first step, but it's not likely to rid kids' lives of soda altogether. Teens, in particular, will buy their own—unless parents begin, from the time their kids are small, to educate them about the hazards of colas.

To build adequate bone in childhood, kids should get an average of 60 minutes of robust physical activity every day. Running, playing soccer, jumping rope, in-line skating and team sports are fun ways to build up bone. Helping with chores around the house and yard helps keep kids active, too, and gives you a break! The Surgeon General reports that *half* of American kids don't do the

An unsuspecting bone robber is "wheat" products such as bread, pasta, and many foods with wheat included in them. Sprue or "Celiacs Disease" as it is known is a serious inability to digest the gluten in grains such as wheat, oats, and barley. One of the side effects can be mild to severe "calcium deficiency." It's not surprising to see blood types "O," "A," & "AB" having difficulty with gluten products also.

minimum amount of ex-
ercise required to keep
their bones fit.

CHEERLEADING INJURIES: WARNING SIGN OF WEAKER BONES IN TEENS

Cheerleading isn't just for
high school gym pep ral-
lies anymore. It's a major
sport, emphatically em-
braced by (mostly) girls
and women. In 2002,
3.5 million kids aged six
and older participated in
cheerleading—an 18 per-
cent increase since 1990.

Along with the in-
crease in number of par-
ticipants has come a sig-
nificant rise in the rate of
injuries. One study
showed a 110 percent in-
crease in the number of
injuries between 1990 and
2002, although the overall
participation in cheerleading increased by only 18 percent. This
study used a national injury database to identify trends in cheer-
leading-related injuries; of the 223,000 cheerleading injuries that
were examined over a 13-year period, 208,800 children between the
ages of five and 18 were hurt badly enough to require treatment at
the emergency room. Children between five and 11 years of age were
more likely to turn up with broken or dislocated bones in response
to these injuries than older children (Children's Hospital 2007).

This heightened number of injuries is a good indication that these girls' bones are not as strong as they need to be. For cheerpersons and all other young girls, calcium with the extra supporting mineral/nutrient supplementation, diet, and strength training may be a big help. You'll learn more about the best supplemental sources of calcium in Chapter 5.

WHAT MEN NEED TO KNOW NOW
ABOUT THEIR BONE HEALTH

Older men fall *more often* than elderly women, according to Dr. Thurman Lockhart of Virginia Polytech Institute (ABC News 2003). Increasingly greater numbers of men are experiencing bone fractures, broken hips and loss of height.

According to Tom Weber, M.D., an endocrinologist at Duke University, "Two million men in this country have osteoporosis. . . . The risk of hip fracture in men will increase by 300 percent by 2050." This increase is steeper than the increase expected in women.

Men who begin to explore ways to get and stay healthy find plenty about how to guard their prostate glands and prevent a heart attack, but male bone health doesn't get much press. "In some ways it's more serious for men," Dr. Weber states in a 2006 issue of *Duke Medical News.* "Several recent studies have shown that men are at higher risk for death following a hip fracture. That risk may be as high as 40 percent within the first year [after] the fracture, when it's on the order of 20 percent for women."

Although men have larger skeletons and their bone loss starts later in life than women, the risk of osteoporosis is still very much an issue. By the age of 60, white men have 25 percent chance of fracturing a hip or other bone in later years.

One of the keys to understanding men's risk of osteoporosis is a gradual decline in production of the hormone testosterone. While estrogen abruptly drops off at menopause, testosterone production declines steadily over decades. While women can lose up to 20 percent of their bone mass in the first five to seven years following menopause as estrogen levels plummet, men can catch up to women in this area by the age of 65 as their testosterone levels slowly decline.

As is the case with women, other factors have an impact on men's bone health: age, heredity, white race, low calcium intake, inadequate exercise, cigarette smoking, alcohol consumption and prolonged exposure to certain bone-robbing medications (particularly, arthritis drugs, anticonvulsants, and antacids) and food choices (too much protein from meat and dairy, too few vegetables, fruits and legumes). Men with kidney disease, lung disease, digestive disorders, or chronically low testosterone levels may experience accelerated bone loss.

All in all, every man, woman and child who has been brought up on the standard Western diet is at risk for osteoporosis. To forestall a major health care emergency, we all need to take appropriate steps to shift our diets, exercise habits, and supplement programs in ways that will promote better bone density.

The Whole Body Bone Building Program is designed to create a lifestyle of bone building habits through:

- The Fast & Easy *Recipes* Rich in Bone Building Foods
- The *Food and Symptom Chart—Identifies nutritional deficiencies & provides the food list that nourish.*
- The *15 Minute Bone Building Exercise Program*-Strengthens Bones—especially those most vulnerable to fractures.

How? You'll find out in the chapters that follow.

Chapter Five

A Stand-Up Diet for Healthy Bones

A *paleopathologist* is a scientist who studies diseases that occurred in people who lived in the distant past. These scientists also study and compare the incidence and progression of diseases in ancient people and modern people. This line of research has come to the same conclusion many times: that people who lived in the very distant past had almost no cancer, almost no diabetes, and almost no osteoporosis.

The first thing one might think when hearing this: *if you get eaten by a saber-toothed tiger or die of some virulent plague before your 30th birthday*—much likelier eventualities in the days before civilization really got swinging—*you're probably not going to end up with osteoporosis!* But the paleopathologist's have a good comeback for this point. They've controlled for age and lifespan factors in these studies of ancient human skeletons. In other words, they've ruled age out as the only explanation for this far lower incidence of certain diseases.

In the end, science has shown that today's ever-rising prevalence of diseases like osteoporosis, type 2 diabetes, and heart disease—so-called "diseases of civilization"—have a lot to do with the ways in which our diets and activity levels have changed since antiquity. According to one analysis, risk of breast cancer in Western women up to age 60 is 100 times that of the risk for women who lived in pre-agricultural times—the days when hunter-gatherer diets were the only option.

Some small pockets of pre-industrial civilization still exist at this writing: Eskimo's who eat almost exclusively fish and marine mammals; African and Australian aborigines; and a few others. These civilizations are of great interest to modern dietary scientists, as they maintain dietary patterns that stand in stark conflict to those of most of the developed world. So, too, are more advanced civilizations that have managed to hold onto traditional ways of eating.

The most interesting thing to these scientists is to see what happens when Western foods and activity patterns begin to creep into the lives of these pre-industrial people. Sometimes this happens when they emigrate to a new country and start to "do as the Romans do," eating fast food and sitting all day. Sometimes it happens when the Western world invades their small corner of the universe.

In Aboriginal communities before the 1970s, diabetes was extremely rare, but today the prevalence of diabetes there is about 10 percent. Diabetes is also on the rapid rise in the Inuit people who live in Alaska and Greenland as they eat more Western foods. Japanese people who move to the U.S. have increases in cancer, diabetes, and obesity within a single generation. African-Americans and Hispanic Americans are both far more vulnerable to these diseases than people of European origin—as they shift quickly to the calorie-dense, sugary, bad-fat-laden diet that Americans have been eating for generations. And although the most distinct changes are rising incidence of heart disease, obesity, diabetes, and high blood pressure, time is bound to bear out increases in osteoporosis with these shifts as well. This is what occurred with my mother Lucy. She grew up on the farm, from a family of 9 and my grand parents lived a long, healthy life working hard and from their gardens. When my mom went to the city and met my father, they had 11 children but their diets changed to the standard American diet and she developed serious heart disease and unfortunately died in my arms at 53 years young.

What's This Protective
Hunter-Gatherer Diet, Anyhow?

With variations depending on the part of the world, it contains wild fruit, nuts, greens, tubers (e.g. potatoes), insects (!), meat and organs from wild animals, fish, marine mammals, and crustaceans. Shifting from this type of diet to one mostly consisting of industrially farmed, nutrient-depleted grains, meat, and dairy and a great deal of heavily processed oil and refined sugar is now known to be a major aspect of the shift from robust good health to chronic disease and discomfort. The former diet is naturally rich in bioavailable minerals, vitamins, and proteins, while the latter is vastly depleted of the nutrients we need for good health.

It's Not Just About Calcium . . .

By now, you're certainly clear that calcium is essential for the maintenance of healthy bones. You recognize that dairy products aren't the only—or even the optimal—source of this nutrient. In this chapter, you'll discover more about additional sources of calcium from plant foods and supplements crafted from specific calcium-rich plant foods.

Calcium adequacy is the tip of the iceberg. Several other corollary nutrients are required for optimal bone building throughout life. Foods that are good for your bones contain these nutrients, and the best-absorbed, best-utilized supplemental sources of calcium also contain some of these nutrients. They're "the total package," because they come from calcium-rich plant foods with which humans have evolved in a symbiotic relationship over millions of years. No chalky horse pill of calcium carbonate can even begin to match these foods in their value to human health!

. . . But You Do Need to Eat a Calcium-Rich Diet . . .

Sadly, a tremendous number of people consume less than half the recommended daily amount of calcium they need to help their bones stay strong. Now that you know that dairy is not your best primary source of this mineral, you're ready to learn about the whole host of non-dairy, whole-food sources of calcium from which you can choose. See the Recipe section for suggestions about how to include these foods in your daily diet.

The situation we're in with calcium could be likened to the hormone replacement therapy scandal of the early 2000s. Calcium supplements are an enormous business, as are dairy foods, and they've cornered the market on bone health. And the Pharmacuetical Industry is right up there also. As you've seen, this could turn out to be disastrous, as consumers load up on these inferior sources of calcium and end up with crumbling bones.

The nutritional research that seems to offer such unequivocal support of the dairy/calcium salts (carbonate, citrates, phosphate, gluconates, coral calcium) approach to bone health has been funded by the same industries that stand to profit from their widespread use. Those who have the money can pay to have studies done that are guaranteed to yield positive results. With regard to dairy calcium and dead calcium salts: who do you believe at this point?

I hope I've been able to show you the core truth on these issues. A hundred years ago, before all this dairy/calcium mineral salt supplement hype, bones were better and stronger. I believe that today, we can return to that place with whole foods rich in calcium and the supporting nutrients with their co-factors, and rarely have a challenge with absorption, utilization and retention of these bone-builders. We can have a better future, and the time for a turnaround is now.

People are buying a lot of calcium salts and taking high doses to try to match U.S. recommendations. How much calcium, then, do you require if you are avoiding bone-robbers and getting regular exercise? Although the U.S. RDA for adult intake of calcium is between 800 and 1200 mg per day (1200 for elderly, 400–800 mg per day for children under the age of four), the World Health Organization's calcium recommendations are 400–500 mg per day. If you practice the Whole Body Bone Building Program by combining these foods with a diet not too high or too low in protein, avoid bone-robbers, and exercise regularly with the fast and energizing program included, include the wonderful foods and recipes included in this book (to order the "Whole Body Bone Building Program" call (888) 456–1597), you don't need to swallow crushed rocks or oyster shells to amp up your intake of this mineral!

Non-Dairy Sources of Calcium	Amount	Calcium (mg)
Oatmeal made with rice milk	1 cup	300
Sardines with bones (no salt)	3 oz.	325
Collards, cooked	1 cup	266
Spinach [OXALATE]	1 cup	291
Salmon with bones (no salt)	3 oz.	180
Bok choi (Chinese cabbage)	1 cup	74
Carrots	1 cup	34
Baked beans	1 cup	154
Peas in pods	1 cup	42
Blackstrap molasses	1 Tbsp.	172
Turnip greens, cooked	½ cup	124
Ocean perch	3 oz.	116
Chickpeas (garbanzo beans), cooked	½ cup	106
Tofu with calcium	3 oz.	30–100
Green or red cabbage	1 cup	42–45
Kale, cooked	1 cup	90
Almonds/almond butter	1 oz.	72
Broccoli, cooked	1 cup	71
Shrimp	3 oz.	45
Other veggies and most fruit	1 cup	10–60

from http://hgic.clemson.edu/factsheets/HGIC4018.htm and the USDA database

Go Organic, Pesticide & Chemical Free!

Unlike dairy products, plant sources of calcium are packed with antioxidant nutrients like carotenes, flavonoids, and selenium—nutrients that protect against free radical damage that is a causal factor in early aging and chronic and degenerative diseases. Plant sources of calcium are also rich in fiber, B vitamins, and minerals, and promote an alkaline, well-oxygenated environment in the body.

Keep in mind, too, that many of the other foods we eat can actually interfere with calcium absorption. For instance, a meat-based, salty meal such as a burger and fries can cause any calcium you have taken in with it to bypass the bones completely and be excreted through urination. And dairy products, although they contain a lot of calcium, contain too much protein to make them a reliable source.

... AND TAKE YOUR CALCIUM SUPPLEMENTS!

For optimal bone nourishment that helps to prevent porous bones, look for a highly absorbable, naturally derived source of calcium and rich in minerals with co-factor nutrients which can only be found in real foods.

HOW ABOUT CALCIUM-FORTIFIED PRODUCTS?

Don't rely on calcium fortification to meet your daily calcium requirements. Fortification uses the same calcium citrates and carbonates that come from chalk, rocks and shells. These substances make a different kind of bone matrix than that built by whole food calcium with all its co-factors. The latter kind of calcium builds intelligent, mineralized bone; the former builds bone that can break and snap like chalk.

Keep in mind that supplements are not monitored or regulated by the Food and Drug Administration the same way prescription drugs are, so you need to be well aware of what to look for when selecting a calcium supplement.

A quick reference list on what to look for:

■ Absolutely look for a whole food supplement that includes the 18 minerals and nutrients with co-factors—the needed nutrients that plant sources of calcium naturally contain.

■ Before purchasing any supplement, be sure you understand the source of the calcium, its rate of absorption, and how much you will require daily to meet your requirements. Some calcium supplements, particularly those made of calcium carbonate or calcium citrate, can increase the risk of developing kidney problems if too much is taken. A plant can absorb them but humans have serious difficulty in doing so.

■ Is the size of the supplement too large to swallow? The daunting task of swallowing a gigantic pill may be enough to cause a person to skip doses. And a huge pill is likely to end up giving you "expensive urine," since only a portion of a high dose can be assimilated at once and the rest is likely to pass out in the urine or lodge in the blood stream. I recommend powdered, chewable or smaller-sized supplements, taken several times each day for maximum utilization and absorbability. Taking the largest amount at night will help relax you into a deep, rejuvenating sleep.

A lifetime with a straight spine and strong bones isn't the only benefit that calcium offers our bodies. Calcium can help lower blood pressure, and may even guard against heart disease and colon cancer. So, the question remains: what are good sources of supplemental whole-food calcium that will help you meet your body's need for plant-based bone nutrition?

A NATURAL, BIO-ABSORBABLE CALCIUM SOURCE: *HYDRILLA VERTICULATA*

In my own explorations, I've discovered some extraordinary calcium sources. One of the best by far is an invasive, fast-growing freshwater plant called *Hydrilla verticulata*.

Native to the warmer areas of Asia, *Hydrilla* has also been found in Europe, Asia, Australia, New Zealand, Africa and South America. *Hydrilla* accumulates high levels of calcium from the calcium-rich soil it thrives in. When dried, the plant's weight is 13 percent calcium.

In the 1960s, this highly adaptive plant was found deeply rooted in the fresh water lakes and streams of Florida where it grows abundantly. It has spread rapidly, and is now found in all Gulf Coast states: off the Atlantic as far north as Maryland and in the Western states including California, Washington and Arizona. In fact, this plant grows so fast and so well that it has thrown many aquatic ecosystems out of balance, requiring remediation—not so good in the natural setting, but an excellent clue as to its potential as a cultivated source of bio-available, plant-sourced calcium.

In addition to its calcium bounty, *Hydrilla* is also rich in proteins, carbohydrates, iron, vitamin B-12 and beta-carotene. It's no wonder that *Hydrilla* has long been popular with vegans who seek out whole-food calcium sources.

From its underwater roots, *Hydrilla's* stems break the water surface, enabling the plant to intercept sunlight and to make efficient use of available nutrients. Because *Hydrilla* tissue is composed of a high percentage of water, it can produce fresh plant material from a limited supply of essential plant nutrients such as carbon, nitrogen and phosphorus.

Hydrilla's complex matrix of bio-absorbable nutrients makes it my top calcium choice. It's alkaline and easily absorbed and delivered to body cells. I'd even go so far as to say that this hardy plant is a gift from the earth.

Seaweeds, in general, are also rich in highly bioavailable calcium. Enjoy kelp, dulse, and nori as condiments or as whole food supplements; use wakame, hijiki, arame, and kombu in soups and stews. Algae-sourced calcium supplements can also be used to fill your calcium requirements, as long as they are whole foods that contain the other nutrients required for absorption and utilization.

NUTRIENTS (WITH CO-FACTORS) YOU NEED WITH YOUR CALCIUM

While many calcium supplements are available, they usually do not contain other bone nutrients (or very few) that work *with* calcium to build strong bones. Robert P. Heaney, M.D., professor of medicine at Creighton University in Omaha, Nebraska, warns: "Bone health isn't just a calcium issue." (Ladies Home Journal 2006).

To complement your calcium intake, seek out real, whole food supplements that contain complementary nutrients which are crucial support and can enhance the absorption of the calcium while supplying the essential nutrient companions needed for strong bones. And the good news is that there's now a promising generation of bone-building nutrients that work together to help halt bone loss.

The 18 Nutrients with Co-Factors: What They Are, What They Do, Where To Get Them

NUTRIENT	WHY IT'S NEEDED FOR BONE HEALTH	SOURCES	OTHER BENEFITS/ POINTS WORTH NOTING
Calcium	It is critical for over 350 different metabolic processes like building teeth & bones, relaxing muscles, regulating such important processes like your metabolism, hormones, heartbeats, nerve impulses, producing insulin, helping you sleep. Even though it is the most abundant mineral—it can't do it alone. It needs the nutrients	Asparagus, Collard Greens, Turnip Greens, Kelp, Dulse, Brocolli, Chlorella, Watercress, Chickpeas, Sesame Seeds, Sunflower Seeds, Burdock Root, Cayenne, Fenugreek, Fennelseed, Chickweed, Nettle, Rose Hips, Yellow Dock, Blackstrap Molasses, Plantain, Water Algae, Hydrilla Verticulatta, Chia Seed, Yucca Root.	Calcium is responsible for the foundation of our bones-the frame of our house-our body. Your alkali reserves originate in your bones and mineralization must be strong to withstand the stresses of everyday life. Poor, acid forming food choices, stress, colas, medications, and wheat can wreak havoc on your bone mineral reserves and thus calcium pours out of the bones to neutralize the acid

The 18 Nutrients with Co-Factors: What They Are, What They Do, Where To Get Them

NUTRIENT	WHY IT'S NEEDED FOR BONE HEALTH	SOURCES	OTHER BENEFITS/ POINTS WORTH NOTING
	below to support its, absorption utilization & retention in the body.		that has occurred. Fill your bone bank daily with mineral rich foods from these charts as well as a good whole food supplement.
Magnesium	Although this mineral gets far less press than calcium, it's important for bone health and cardio-vascular health. It participates in over 300 metabolic reactions that produce energy and build tissues (including bone) within the body.	Kelp, apple pectin fiber, apricots, ba-nana, brown rice, blackstrap molasses, dulse, garlic, lemon, black-eyed peas, cantaloupe, lima beans, wa-tercress, blad-derwrack, cay-enne, red clover, yellow dock, chia seed.	Magnesium also helps reduce in-flammation and allergic reactions. Migraine, diabetes, hypertension, al-lergies, asthma, cramping, twitch-ing, arrythmias and even depression. agoraphobia & anxiety have been linked with low in-take. Synthetic: ci-trate, gluconate, or oxide. They dehy-drate the body, pull-ing liquid into the stomach and often cause diarrhea/soft stools. Can deplete minerals.

The 18 Nutrients with Co-Factors: What They Are, What They Do, Where To Get Them

NUTRIENT	WHY IT'S NEEDED FOR BONE HEALTH	SOURCES	OTHER BENEFITS/ POINTS WORTH NOTING
Vitamin K	A protein called osteocalcin serves as a "glue" that helps incorporate calcium into bone. Vitamin K—in particular, the form of this vitamin known as K2—is needed for the action of this protein.	A single one-cup serving of raw kale contains about five times the adult RDA of vitamin K; a cup of spinach contains just over the RDA; a cup of Swiss chard or a cup of broccoli contain twice the RDA. Two forms of vitamin K exist: K1 and K2. More on this in the section on vitamin K on page 138.	A deficiency of vitamin K is one of the risk factors for osteoporosis—and for calcification of arteries, a problem linked with heart attack and stroke. Vitamin K plays a role as calcium "gatekeeper," helping to dictate whether calcium moves into the bones or into the soft lining of blood vessels. Vitamin K also helps to promote heart health by aiding in blood coagulation. (Because it's a pro-clotting nutrient, people taking blood thinners such as Coumadin are advised to avoid it.)

The 18 Nutrients with Co-Factors: What They Are, What They Do, Where To Get Them

NUTRIENT	WHY IT'S NEEDED FOR BONE HEALTH	SOURCES	OTHER BENEFITS/ POINTS WORTH NOTING
Phosphorus	Next to calcium, phosphorous is the most abundant mineral in the body. These two minerals work in synch to build strong bones and teeth. In fact, 85 percent of phosphorous in the body is located in bones and teeth; the remaining amount channels through cells and tissues, helping to repair them.	Asparagus, garlic, sesame, pumpkin seeds. A good whole-food calcium supplement will contain balancing phosphorus.	It is this action that helps the body to recover from muscle pain after a hard workout. Phosphorous also helps to escort waste out of the kidneys and aids in breaking down carbohydrates, protein and fats. This mineral also helps the body to balance and metabolize other vitamins and minerals, including calcium, vitamin D, magnesium and zinc. The human body can become phosphorous-deficient when exposed to an excessive intake of aluminum-containing substances such as antacids. Diabetes, Crohn's disease and alcoholism can con-

The 18 Nutrients with Co-Factors: What They Are, What They Do, Where To Get Them

NUTRIENT	WHY IT'S NEEDED FOR BONE HEALTH	SOURCES	OTHER BENEFITS/ POINTS WORTH NOTING
			tribute to the body's weakened ability to absorb nutrients which drains the body's phosphorous levels.
Vitamin B3 (niacin)	This B vitamin is required for cellular energy production, DNA repair, and cellular communication. It helps to maintain the health of skin and joints.	Peanuts and other nuts, fish, potatoes, whole grains, broccoli, burdock root, cayenne, fennel seed, nettle, red clover, rose hips, wild yam.	Niacin interacts with other nutrients to promote overall health— cardiovascular, skin, skeletal, joint, and immune.

The 18 Nutrients with Co-Factors: What They Are, What They Do, Where To Get Them

NUTRIENT	WHY IT'S NEEDED FOR BONE HEALTH	SOURCES	OTHER BENEFITS/ POINTS WORTH NOTING
Vitamin B6	Vitamin B6 is important in bone metabolism as it is a co-factor which promotes linking collagen strands and strengthening connective tissue in bones, needed for creating HCI production for digesting and absorption of calcium, helps adrenal function for the best mineralization.	Found in Brown Rice, Soybeans, wheat germ, butter, fish, meat, whole grain cereals.	Helps break down homocysteine which interferes with the collagen cross linking which can create a defective bone matrix resulting in osteoporosis. Hip fracture sufferers often test low in Vit. B6. B6 is important to break down fats, proteins, and carbohydrates thus it is critical for the liver processes also. Too much B6 as a synthetic supplement has been linked to poor sense of touch, nerve damage, numbness, tingling, impaired walking.

The 18 Nutrients with Co-Factors: What They Are, What They Do, Where To Get Them

NUTRIENT	WHY IT'S NEEDED FOR BONE HEALTH	SOURCES	OTHER BENEFITS/ POINTS WORTH NOTING
Lysine	An essential amino acid (protein building block) that's turning out to be important for bone strength. It appears to help the body to absorb calcium and build collagen, the matrix upon which bone, skin, and all other connective tissue is built.	Lima beans, fish, nuts, eggs, soybeans, spirulina, fenugreek seed. Lysine is responsible in part for the browning that occurs when flour products are baked or fried, this process binds the sugars to lysine permanently & makes them unabsorbable.	*Lysine* is needed to make another amino acid called carnitine. Carnitine, in turn, converts fats in the body into energy, reducing the amount of fat floating around in the bloodstream in the form of triglycerides. This is good news for heart health. A diet with adequate lysine is also helpful for prevention of herpes virus and shingles outbreaks.
Zinc	Zinc has been shown to stimulate bone formation and inhibit bone loss in multiple animal studies Critical for bone	Oysters and other shellfish, legumes (especially pinto beans, black-eyed peas, soybeans, peanuts), pumpkin seeds, whole grains,	Zinc also has antioxidant effects, and plays roles in immunity, appetite, stress response, taste, smell, normal growth and development, reproduction. Typical

The 18 Nutrients with Co-Factors: What They Are, What They Do, Where To Get Them

NUTRIENT	WHY IT'S NEEDED FOR BONE HEALTH	SOURCES	OTHER BENEFITS/ POINTS WORTH NOTING
	healing, enhances biochemical activy of Vit. D. A deficiency prevents full calcium absorb.	miso, tofu, brewer's yeast, cooked greens, mushrooms, green beans, tahini, and sun-flower seeds.	U.S. adults only consume 2/3 of the RDA.
Silicon	Silica is critical to bone health, helping the body to process minerals such as iron, calcium, magnesium, potassium and boron. Many believe that silicon may be just as potent in strengthening a human's musculoskeletal system as it is in keeping the giant elephant's skeletal system fluid and durable.	Bamboo, celery, Boston and Bibb lettuces. Oat straw and horsetail silica, the more popu-lar forms of this supplement, are only eight percent silica; bamboo silica supplements can contain as much as 85 percent silica. While the In-dian elephant is smaller than its African cousin, it is much, much stronger. What gives this	Getting adequate silicon can help beautify and strengthen nails, hair, and skin as well as carry miner-als and nutrients into the bones for strengthening the bones. It does this by strengthening the connective tis-sue matrix via cross linking the protein-collagen strands.

The 18 Nutrients with Co-Factors: What They Are, What They Do, Where To Get Them

NUTRIENT	WHY IT'S NEEDED FOR BONE HEALTH	SOURCES	OTHER BENEFITS/ POINTS WORTH NOTING
	This mineral promotes the formation of collagen (the basic building block of all connective tissue, including bone, skin, and cartilage) and bone mineralization.	smaller mammal its incredibly strong, yet flexible, skeletal system? Experts believe it comes from the elephant's principal diet of bamboo.	
Vitamin C	This vitamin is needed for the formation of collagen, which is the protein matrix upon which bone is built. It also promotes better calcium absorption. Getting enough C can actually make bone denser; promising studies show vitamin C	Peruvian Camu Camu fruit, Amla fruit, Rose hips, acerola, goji berries, acai, pomagranate fruit and inner skin, sea buckthorn, jujube (the herb, not the candy!), black currant, carrots, strawberry fruit, red peppers, parsley, guava, kiwi fruit, citrus	Many animals manufacture their own vitamin C. Goats, for example, make the equivalent of 13,000 mg per day—a much higher relative dose than humans are advised to obtain daily. This antioxidant nutrient, which promotes great immunity, which helps reduce inflammation and asthma symptoms,

The 18 Nutrients with Co-Factors: What They Are, What They Do, Where To Get Them

NUTRIENT	WHY IT'S NEEDED FOR BONE HEALTH	SOURCES	OTHER BENEFITS/ POINTS WORTH NOTING
	can reverse osteoporosis in lab animals. Vit. C promotes the production of adrenal hormones needed for gd bones	fruits, brussels sprouts, elderberry, persimmon.	may be like vitamin D in that we underestimate our need for it in whole-food form.
Manganese	This mineral is an important constitutent of several kinds of enzymes in the body, and catalyzes the reactions of other enzymes as well. Deficiency is linked to abnormal bone development; one of the enzymes it catalyzes is necessary for proper formation of	Dulse, seaweed, blueberries, pineapple, burdock root, fennel seed, fenugreek, rose hips, wild yam, yellow dock, almonds, pecans, oatmeal, peanuts, other legumes. Daily amounts may be more than 2 mg (3 to 7 mg) as calcium, iron, phosphorous and zinc can reduce manganese absorption.	Also important for wound healing and good liver cleansing function. Manganese lack is also more likely in people with diabetes. Pro basketball player Bill Walton's chronic bone injury's popularized the need for this mineral as it is critical for bone collagen and cartilage formation as well as proper bone metabolism. Deficiency increases not only bone break-

The 18 Nutrients with Co-Factors: What They Are, What They Do, Where To Get Them

NUTRIENT	WHY IT'S NEEDED FOR BONE HEALTH	SOURCES	OTHER BENEFITS/ POINTS WORTH NOTING
	bone. Studies suggest that women with osteoporosis have lower manganese levels and respond more strongly to supplementation.		down but decreases remineralization of the bones.
"Vitamin F"— essential fats	Several studies suggest that omega-3 fats promote better skeletal growth. Studies of blood levels of fatty acids show that higher levels of these fats are correlated with better bone mineral density.	Flax seeds, acai, goji, fatty fish like salmon, borage oil, primrose oil, chia seeds.	The average American diet is very low on omega-3s and high in far less healthful omega-6 fats. Shifting this ratio may improve immune, psychological, and cardiovascular health a great deal.
Vitamin D	Unlike other vitamins, this one can be made in the body, and it acts like a	Sun exposure, egg yolk, fish liver oils, fish, chlorella ("liquid sunshine"),	Vitamin D also plays a role in maintaining the immune system and in regulat-

The 18 Nutrients with Co-Factors: What They Are, What They Do, Where To Get Them

NUTRIENT	WHY IT'S NEEDED FOR BONE HEALTH	SOURCES	OTHER BENEFITS/ POINTS WORTH NOTING
	hormone, in that it sends a message to the small intestinal wall, where bone-building minerals are absorbed. Its message: "Allow plenty of calcium and phosphorus through into the bloodstream." This message is directly linked to the level of mineralization that occurs in the bones. Low levels can lead to overactive parathyroid thus promoting bone loss. Eighty percent of elderly hip fractures were low in vitamin D.	nettle, white button mushrooms (see the Sidebar, below). New research shows osteoporosis can be stopped and you can actually increase bone mass in the winter with with appropriate vitamin D & calcium.	ing healthy cell growth—both elements of cancer protection. Low vitamin D levels have also been linked to osteomalacia (pre-osteoporosis softening of the bones), increased risk of breast, colon, and prostate cancers, diabetes, epilepsy, seasonal depression, bipolar disorder, and even schizophrenia. People who live in places that get a lot of sun have lower incidence of cancer than those who live in sunny areas, and obese people have lower levels of vitamin D—possibly, this could help explain the link between obesity and most cancers.

The 18 Nutrients with Co-Factors: What They Are, What They Do, Where To Get Them

NUTRIENT	WHY IT'S NEEDED FOR BONE HEALTH	SOURCES	OTHER BENEFITS/ POINTS WORTH NOTING
Chromium picolinate	This mineral helps to maintain good blood sugar balance by potentiating the blood sugar-lowering effects of insulin. In doing so, it may help prevent glucose intolerance and type 2 diabetes—which, in turn, may help prevent osteoporosis.	Brown rice, blackstrap molasses, red clover, wild yam, broccoli, grape juice.	Although claims that chromium helps build muscle haven't panned out in the research, some research evidence indicates that it can help slow weight gain in people who are insulin resistant.
Folate (synthetic form is folic acid)	A few studies suggest that high levels of a substance called *homocysteine* may be linked to osteoporosis. Folic acid, a B vitamin, is needed to keep homocysteine levels low. This condition is associated with heart disease.	The word "folate" comes from the word *foliage,* and for good reason: green leafy vegetables are the best source. Others: cantaloupe, brewer's yeast, oranges, bananas, red fruits, nuts, avocados, whole grains.	Folate is needed for normal cellular growth and maintenance. Dangerous folate depletion can be created by pregnancy, alcoholism, and a long list of drugs, including anticonvulsants, methotrexate, trimethoprim, triamterene, and sulfasalazine.

The 18 Nutrients with Co-Factors: What They Are, What They Do, Where To Get Them

NUTRIENT	WHY IT'S NEEDED FOR BONE HEALTH	SOURCES	OTHER BENEFITS/ POINTS WORTH NOTING
B12	Helps make the red blood cells in our bodies and is stored in our livers.	Found in egg yolk, meat, liver, and poultry.	B12 is needed for proper function of the osteoblasts which build new bone cells. The amount needed may be much higher than once thought of 3 mcg.
Boron	This mineral converts vitamin D into its active form and helps maintain calcium, magnesium and phosphorous balance. We require two milligrams a day. It's found most abundantly in vegetables and fruit, which helps explain why many Americans don't get enough.	Apples, grapes, cilantro, collard greens, broccoli	Most boron supplements come from boric acid, which is used to kill roaches. Choose a plant-sourced, whole-food bone-building supplement to get a form that is well-absorbed and used by the body. A plant source comes from a plant.

The 18 Nutrients with Co-Factors: What They Are, What They Do, Where To Get Them

NUTRIENT	WHY IT'S NEEDED FOR BONE HEALTH	SOURCES	OTHER BENEFITS/ POINTS WORTH NOTING
Protein	You need adequate protein in your diet to properly assimilate calcium. The form of calcium is the challenge. Using non plant sources (meat, fish, poultry) can cause acidosis (high acidity and low oxygenation) in the body which is linked to degenerative disease.	Fortunately, almost no American needs to worry about getting enough protein. We get more than enough; see page 46 for more on this. Excellent vegetarian sources include hemp, quinoa and other grains, nuts, nut butters, legumes, yellow pea, brown rice, spirulina (which has more protein than meat at 65 percent protein).	With all of the problems that are fed by meat as protein source—bird flu, mad cow, pollution, hormones, high concentration of toxins—it's high time we recognize that we can build muscle, stay lean, and avoid chronic disease without meat. Even fish is becoming more contaminated; you are best off with wild fish.

Additional Useful Information
on Co-factor Nutrients

Magnesium

Magnesium helps reduce inflammation and allergic reactions. Migraine, osteoporosis, diabetes, hypertension, allergies, asthma, and even depression and anxiety have been linked with low intake of magnesium. Magnesium is so important that no fewer than three scientific journals have been created to publish research on this mineral.

Humans evolved in an environment extremely rich in magnesium—it's the eighth most plentiful element in the earth's crust and the third most plentiful element in ocean water. At the center of each molecule of chlorophyll, the green pigment in plants that enables them to make their own food from sunlight, is magnesium. Of the roughly 25 grams found in the body of an adult human, 60 percent is incorporated into bone. The rest is found in muscle and circulating around in the bloodstream and elsewhere.

A link between magnesium deficiency and osteoporosis has long been suspected, and now research is confirming this possibility: scientists at Tel Aviv University in Israel, for example, have induced osteoporosis in rats by depleting them of magnesium long-term.

In another study, one group of menopausal women got intravenous infusions of magnesium regularly for two years, and had higher bone mineral density (BMD) in the end than did women who did not get the IV magnesium; and in yet another study, menopausal women on a high-magnesium diet had gains in BMD compared to menopausal women who were not on this diet. This study suggests that long-term lack of magnesium may be made up for, at least in part, with high-dose infusions of this mineral. With this kind of approach, however, we could be setting ourselves up for problems like bone spurs, which is sometimes seen with high-dose coral calcium, carbonates, and citrates given to make up for a lifetime of calcium lack.

Magnesium is most abundant in foods that have not been subjected to processing. Turning whole grain into white bread strips it of most of its magnesium. Dry beans, chlorella, split peas, leafy greens, avocado, shrimp, and clams are excellent dietary sources of this mineral.

As it turns out, most of us don't get enough of it in our diets—according to some experts, 80 percent of Americans aren't meeting the bare-bones requirement for this calming, heartbeat-regulating mineral. (The RDA is 420 mg for men, 310 mg for women, and 350 mg for pregnant women.) This deficiency is made worse yet by the widespread popping of high-dose calcium pills, which reduce retention of magnesium in the body. According to magnesium researcher Mildred Seelig, Ph.D., too much calcium relative to magnesium can predispose us to dangerous blood clots. Magnesium reduces the "stickiness" of blood clots, making them less dangerous. Magnesium rich plant foods can be beneficial to reverse this condition.

A worthwhile goal: to consume real, whole food supplements and foods that contain the proper ratio of calcium to magnesium—about two to one. (Hydrilla, a source of calcium (I'll touch upon later in this chapter), contains this ratio of calcium and magnesium.) This isn't too hard to do when you get these nutrients from whole food sources, where they naturally exist in the appropriate ratio.

When estrogen levels drop after menopause, magnesium's ability to build bone can be adversely affected. It's especially important to maintain an adequate intake of this mineral during these years.

How to add more magnesium to one's daily diet? For a magnesium-rich meal, pile fresh raw leafy baby greens on a plate, mixed with chopped baby bok choi, collard greens, or mustard greens, on a plate, then top with avocado, raw cashews, and other chopped vegetables. Shrimp and brown rice can add magnesium to this mix. Top with a dressing made with creamy soft tofu (see Recipes) to add calcium.

If you take a calcium supplement, make sure it's a whole food supplement, and that you're getting about half as much magnesium as calcium daily. If you have a lot of symptoms of magnesium deficiency—listed in the Sidebar—you may want to take it in a 1:1 ratio for a few weeks before shifting back to the 2:1 ratio for which we're designed. Take the whole food magnesium away from the whole food calcium supplement until your symptoms disappear.

Synthetic forms of magnesium will *exacerbate those problems*, including bone loss and decreased calcium utilization. Don't go there!

Avoid magnesium oxide, citrate, and gluconate, which are mineral salts that cake in your stomach, steal your hydration and when combined in the stomach, it creates a "chemical reaction" like a drug does, thus causing a stool softening or diarrhea like effect. It's easy to get hooked on those fizzy, lemony, berry drinks as they help you go the bathroom & seem to calm you initially but research shows that the only way to resolve a magnesium deficiency is through the real, live foods on the list. Research even suggests that these synthetic supplements can leave you more deficient than before.

Vitamin D

Without adequate vitamin D, the absorption of calcium is minimized. This is because vitamin D acts as an escort for calcium, helping to guide it deep into the bones. The moment sunlight kisses the skin, vitamin D production kicks into gear. Some vitamin

Complementary medicine physician Sidney Baker, M.D. describes the symptoms of magnesium deficiency as follows. Most are linked to reduced relaxation of muscle, both skeletal (the voluntary muscles that move the body around) and smooth (the involuntary muscles of the heart, blood vessel walls, and intestinal tract):

A lump in the throat
Agoraphobia
Anxiety, panic attacks
Backache, neck pain, tension headache, jaw tightness or TMJ
Carbohydrate cravings
Chest tightness, inability to take a deep breath, frequent sighing
Constipation
Difficulty adjusting vision when going from dark to light
Difficulty swallowing
Heart palpitations/arrhythmias
Hyperactivity
Insomnia
Loud noise sensitivity
Menstrual cramps or premenstrual irritability, breast tenderness
Muscle twitches, cramps, tension, soreness
Numbness, tingling, and other abnormal sensations—zipping, vibratory sensations
Restlessness
Salt cravings (yet intolerant to it)
Urinary spasms

D is stored in your liver and body fat during the summer, and is released in the winter as required by the body.

According to research published in the *American Journal of Clinical Nutrition,* the commonly recommended daily dose of 800 to 1,000 IU of vitamin D isn't adequate for prevention of osteoporosis. This study was what's known as a *meta-analysis,* where many studies on the same subject are grouped to get a big-picture snapshot. Eighteen studies involving 57,311 participants were grouped, and the researchers concluded that from 2,000 up to 10,000 IU—far above the RDA—may be most effective.

It seems that vitamin D recommendations are going in the same direction as recommendations for daily calcium intake: up, up, and away. Studies that support high-dose synthetic nutrient therapy for disease prevention are still barking up the wrong tree but with Vitamin D though-the current dosage needs clarification.

Research suggests that doses of vitamin D currently recommended are far, far *below* those that were once consumed and created through sun exposure. Keep in mind that 1 million IU's (international units)of vitamin D is equal to 1 single mg (milligram)! To be focusing on 400 to 800 IU's just may not make the best sense. Vitamin D deficiency has been linked with numerous, very serious health challenges and setting the nutritional values at such low IU's seems ridiculous when you put things in perspective. So it makes sense, at this point, to look at much higher doses of *natural sources* of Vitamin D.

Embroiled in this perfect storm of osteoporosis risk factors: increasing use of sunscreen, which blocks out the same ultraviolet rays that stimulate the production of calcium supporter vitamin D in the skin. Total sun blockade has been advised as

---

SUNBATHED MUSHROOMS AN EXCELLENT SOURCE OF VITAMIN D

Although mushrooms are grown in the dark, researchers have found that exposing them to even five minutes' worth of ultraviolet light (either with special lamps indoors, or in sunlight outdoors) after harvesting will increase their vitamin D content to some 869 percent of the RDA—twice as much as is found in a tablespoon of cod liver oil, previously believed to be an optimal source.

a protective barrier against UV-induced skin cancer. Even children are being draped, slathered, and shaded against sunshine with increasing urgency as well-meaning parents try to protect them against sunburn, skin aging and skin cancer. Unfortunately, this may also deprive them of adequate vitamin D, the "sunshine vitamin."

Without adequate vitamin D, the absorption of calcium is minimized. This is because vitamin D acts as an escort for calcium, helping to guide it deep into the bones. The moment sunlight kisses the skin, vitamin D production kicks into gear. Some vitamin D is stored in your liver and body fat during the summer, and is released in the winter as required by the body.

More and more studies are demonstrating that many people, especially seniors and those who live in northern latitudes, aren't getting enough vitamin D to protect their bones. One study performed in Baltimore indicated that up to 60 percent of seniors over the age of 65 were vitamin D deficient, leaving them extremely vulnerable to weak bones, falls and fractures. (Dreifus 2003) The same appears true for teens: in one study performed on Boston teenagers who seemed completely healthy at their regular checkups, nearly ¼ turned out to be deficient in vitamin D. This problem is more prevalent in children with dark skin than in Caucasians, who more easily absorb sunshine into their skin to make vitamin D.

Obesity and advancing age also conspire to reduce vitamin D levels in the body. Crohn's disease, gluten intolerance, cystic fibrosis, gastric bypass (stomach-stapling surgery), medications that reduce fat absorption into the body, or steroid drugs will all reduce vitamin D in the body.

Another potential effect of long-term vitamin D lack: chronic pain. Gregory Plotnikoff, M.D., was practicing medicine at an inner-city primary care clinic, and had encountered 150 patients with persistent muscular and skeletal pain. These were poor people, who had been through a medical boondoggle as they tried to find relief. Some had had extensive medical tests—even were referred to mental health services because of their insistence that they were in pain despite no discernable physical cause.

When he began to investigate, he found that European researchers had been examining this relationship for over three decades. There, studies had found severe vitamin D deficiency in immigrant women who had been suffering chronic musculoskeletal pain. Dr. Plotnikoff tested these patients, who were of six different ethnicities and ranged in age from 10 to 65, for vitamin D deficiency. *Ninety-three percent* were deficient in this vitamin, and 100 percent of those who had dark skin were deficient.

Although this study didn't include treating these folks with vitamin D to see whether they improved, subsequent studies have found that high-dose D does relieve musculoskeletal pain in people whose D levels are low. Dr. Plotnikoff gives his patients 50,000 IU of vitamin D twice a week until their levels normalize. (Do NOT, under any circumstances, attempt to do this on your own, without laboratory proof of deficiency; this is a potentially toxic dose for someone who is not deficient. Especially if it is a synthetic form of vitamin D.)

Other interesting research indicates a link between vitamin D deficiency and osteoarthritis. Over 10 percent of people 60 and up have joint pain and deterioration from this disease. In 500 people enrolled in a study at Boston University, those who took in less vitamin D than they needed had three times the risk of developing osteoarthritis compared to those who got the RDA or more. Why would this be? The researchers concluded that lack of vitamin D might alter the shape of bones just enough to change the way they articulate with one another, leading to increased wear and tear.

It's said that taking in more vitamin D from fortified dairy products is a good way to circumvent the need for sunshine. However: the *synthetic* vitamin D used to fortify dairy has been linked with higher risk of overdose and resulting hypercalcemia (too-high levels of calcium in the blood). You *can't* overdose with vitamin D from sunshine, or from whole plant foods. You *can* overdose from fish liver oils (see below).

The RDA for vitamin D is 200 IU for children and adults up to age 50 and 400 IU for those aged 51–70; after 70, it's 600 IU. Whole food sources of vitamin D include egg yolk (20 IU per yolk) and fatty fish like mackerel, salmon, or tuna (250 to 345 IU per serving). Some people choose to take cod liver oil to boost vitamin D. If you do this, you probably don't need to take it daily, as you can store vitamin D in your liver for (literally) a rainy day. Your health care practitioner can help you decide whether or how much of this whole-food form of vitamin D is a good idea for you.

The best way to get your vitamin D without any risk of toxicity: 10 minutes of direct sunlight exposure daily. You needn't expose your skin during the peak hours of 10 and four p.m., when UV rays are strongest.

This is especially crucial for teens. Since about 35 percent of adult bone mass is formed during the years between 13 and 19, kids living in the northeastern U.S. and other places with little sunshine are at greatly increased risk of vitamin D deficiency. One study in the northeast of kids aged six to 21 found that 55 percent had low blood vitamin D levels—and that 90 percent of African-Americans in this group were deficient. A British study found that 70 percent of teen girls were vitamin D deficient.

Boron

This mineral converts vitamin D into its active form and helps maintain calcium, magnesium and phosphorous balance. We require two to three milligrams a day. It's found most abundantly in vegetables and fruit, which helps explain why many Americans don't get enough. One study of postmenopausal women found that supplementing only three milligrams per day of boron caused levels of estradiol and testosterone to rise. Both of these hormones build bone.

In a report published in *Progress in Food and Nutrition Science*, the Australian researchers highlight a study conducted with postmenopausal women. Within eight days of boron supplementation, the participants excreted less calcium and less magnesium. The researchers concluded that "the findings suggest that boron is beneficial for optimal calcium metabolism and in the prevention of bone loss which occur in older women." (Naghii 1993).

Silicon

This mineral promotes the formation of collagen (the basic building block of all connective tissue, including bone, skin, and cartilage) and bone mineralization. While the Indian elephant is smaller than its African cousin, it is much, much stronger. What gives this smaller mammal its incredibly strong, yet flexible, skeletal system? Experts believe it comes from the elephant's principal diet of bamboo, an edible grass that mammals have survived on for thousands of years. Bamboo extract happens to be the richest known source of natural, organic silica, which comprises up to 70 percent of this fast-growing plant. Horsetail and oatstraw silica (about 8 percent silica) have proven to be carriers. They help carry hydration and minerals and other nutrients into the bones thus being known to help make bones stronger.

Silica is the second most abundant element on earth. This essential nutrient plays a starring role in *maintaining* the integrity of the skin (think about how dense and durable an elephant's skin is), ligaments, tendons and bone. The human body is constantly metabolizing silicic acid and eliminating it through urination, hair loss and nail trimming. Foods rich in silica—it's most concentrated in parts of food we usually discard, including the skins of veggies and fruit and the stringy parts of mangoes, celery, and asparagus—allow us to replace what's lost through these routes. That's why when we juice with these foods, we often get rich amounts of silica from the parts we wouldn't originally eat.

On average, at any given time, the body contains 20 grams of silica. However, with age, less silica is absorbed by the body (or do we eat less of these wonderful foods?). With silica loss the signs of premature aging may begin to show with drier, more wrinkled skin, loss of sheen in hair and weak, brittle nails.

Silica is critical to bone health, helping the body to process minerals such as iron, calcium, magnesium, potassium and boron. Many believe that silicon may be just as potent in strengthening a human's musculoskeletal system as it is in keeping the giant elephant's skeletal system fluid and durable.

Finding a whole food supplement with bamboo silica brings an amazing, natural complement into the human body; its silicon is easily and readily absorbed and incorporated into connective tissues. Clearly, bamboo silica is an essential part of the nutrient and mineral combination that bones need to remain strong and pliable through each decade of life—a whole-food source of this important mineral.

Vitamin K

Vitamin K was discovered in the 1930's by a Denmark researcher and was named after the Danish word "koagulation," because it helps your blood coagulate when bleeding, or just to clot properly. Vitamin K assists an enzyme to convert the chemical structure of particular proteins to their mature form, allowing the proteins to bind with calcium. It also activates at least 3 different proteins critical to bone health. Similar to Vitamin D, your body can produce its own Vitamin K from bacteria found naturally in the intestinal tract rather than getting it from the sun like vitamin D. Even so, we need to get vitamin K from our food as most people don't get enough of it according to work done at the Vitamin K Laboratory at Tuft's University. (U.S. Dept. of Agriculture's Human Nutrition Research Center)

Several forms of this vitamin are found in foods, and some are better absorbed and utilized in the body than others. K1, or phylloquinone, is found in green plants—particularly, the green leafy sort. K2 is also known as menaquinone, and it's made in the digestive tract by the "friendly" probiotic bacte-

---

A NOTE ABOUT FILLERS AND ADDITIVES

Health journalist Mike Adams makes a good point in his article on fillers and additives commonly used in standard nutritional supplements ("Vitamin Warning! Some nutritional supplements use hydrogenated oils as fillers," posted at www.naturalnews.com on October 13, 2005): that pharmaceutical companies, whose interest is mainly in the bottom line, make supplements too—because people are catching on to their value, and there's a lot of money to be made. But these big companies have no qualms about using additives and fillers that may be harmful to your health; after all, they use these same additives and fillers to make prescription drugs.

Avoid any supplement that contains artificial colorings or fillers aside from guar gum, vegetable lubricants, silica, and food glaze which are totally natural.

ria that reside there. This form of K is also found in fermented foods like natto (a form of fermented soy).

Vitamin K Food Forms: Spinach (an OXALATE though), kale, broccoli, asparagus, lettuce, cabbage among a few common ones.

THIS IS YOUR BONES ON WHOLE-FOOD BONE-BUILDING DIET AND SUPPLEMENTS

Let's say a paleopathologist of the future were to investigate the bones of people who lived between the 1950s and 2010. What might they find?

Hopefully, they'll see that although we lost track of the right foods for bone strength and health for a time, we got back on track when we realized how much harm a junk-food, vegetable-poor diet and inactivity was doing to our bones. Maybe the anthropologists of the future will find evidence of great big farms where bok choi, kale, collard greens, vitamin D rich mushrooms and chlorella, plantains, gogi berry's, sesame seeds, asparagus, carrots, fennel seed, fenugreek herb, chickweed, and water plants like *hydrilla verticulata and sea vegetables,* bamboo, and other needed mineral rich vegetables and fruits were grown to provide the nourishment we needed and make nourishing whole-food meals and real mineral supplements. Better yet: perhaps those farms will still be operating a few hundred years from now!

Chapter Six

Exercise Curbs Bone Loss
THE WHOLE BODY BONE BUILDING PROGRAM

If you've always been active, good for you . . . and your bones! Even though aging will naturally cause some density loss, your bones are less likely to become brittle enough to break if you slip and fall.

For those who have been lax in maintaining good exercise habits, it's never too late to take preventative measures to build stronger bones to carry you through your life. Even if you begin late in life, exercise will help you to increase muscle strength and improve balance, which will help you to avoid falls in the future. And current evidence shows that it's never too late to build bone density with exercise.

A commitment to daily or almost-daily exercise will also help to make everyday tasks and activities less taxing. A consistent exercise regimen will not only benefit your bones and improve your health— it will also bring you increased energy, enhanced mood, a slimmer waistline and an overall better outlook on life. And the younger you start, the better.

CHILDREN AND YOUNG ADULTS AND EXERCISE

Children should begin exercising before they reach adolescence, since bone mass increases during puberty, reaching its peak between the ages of 20 and 30. Young children will almost always engage in intensely physical play for hours each day if given the opportunity; all adults need do is provide a safe space for this kind of play and let the child go at it. When space is limited or weather doesn't permit outdoor play, caregivers may find it beneficial to lead kids in some sort of indoor fitness activity. Put on music and dance; set up an obstacle course; or pull out the Chinese jump rope or a mini-trampoline. The bouncier the exercise, the better for the child's bones. Most importantly: *set the example for your children!* When they see Mom or Dad working out regularly, they will imitate you—joyfully and willingly hopefully.

Teens tend to start making choices that are bad for bone health—and exercise is no exception. Parents who want to work against these habits can insist that the teen play at least one sport or engage in regular workouts. Help the teen find an activity that's fun for him or her: hip-hop dance, ballet, hockey, gymnastics, soccer, basketball, skateboarding—all will help build bones. Set a good example—you might even make workout time the time you spend with your teen.

Some studies suggest that regular exercise may help develop bone mass in teenagers more effectively than high calcium intake. (The studies in question use calcium salts or dairy calcium, not whole-food plant sources; it may be with the research we are seeing that the absolute best equation is plenty of plant-sourced calcium plus regular exercise.) For teens, exercises involving high-intensity jumping, such as basketball, are extremely beneficial to bone strengthening in young children. Weight lifting is also an important part of teen and young adult fitness and bone health. If all goes well, a healthy teen who stays active can increase bone density by as much as two to eight percent per year.

Middle Age Through "The Change"— Use It Or Lose It

Obviously, an exercise regimen is something to maintain throughout middle age. It's not easy, but it should be a priority, because you can keep building bone at your highest rate through your mid-thirties.

Fast-forward to "the change"—a period during which bone loss may accelerate. During this time, women have a great deal to gain with regular exercise. Menopausal women who took part in a supervised exercise program for two years as part of a study in Germany experienced generally stable bone density, improved strength, and a dip in blood fats. A placebo group that did not change its lifestyle had a decline in bone health and strength and no improvement in blood fats. (Norton, Reuters Health 2004). Let's not forget that exercise is crucial for prevention of heart disease, as well—a malady that is the #1 killer of women.

All age groups—toddler through centurian!—have a lot to gain from exercising at least three times a week. Not only are you taking steps to reduce your risk of osteoporotic fracture and strengthening muscles to help prevent falls; you are also reducing your risk of virtually every disease that sickens and kills aging Americans—including heart disease, cancer, diabetes, and Alzheimer's disease. Regular exercise promotes better immune function, boosts mood (some studies show that consistent workouts are just as effective as antidepressants in this regard) and quells anxiety. All in all, regular workouts are terrific medicine for your quality of life.

Many different activities can provide your bones with the challenge they need to be-

LEAN ON ME: WHY WEIGHT-BEARING EXERCISE IS STRONG-BODY EXERCISE

Swimming is great; so is cycling. But neither of these will build bone adequately, because they don't pit the musculature of legs, hips, and ankles against the powerful force of gravity. **This opposition between the force of muscle, sinew, and bone and the tug of gravity is the key to effective bone building.** It's the call of the environment in which we live to the resources of the body: *stay strong—you're needed!* It's adaptation in action.

Your body is an exquisitely efficient machine; it only allocates energy where needed. And if you sit on your rear and fail to engage in physical activity, your body won't put in the energy to maintain muscle and bone. In other words: use it, or lose it.

Fortunately, once you lose it, if you use it again, you can regain lost muscle and bone mass. So it's never too late to get back into an exercise program—or to get into one for the very first time.

come stronger. The goal, when it comes to bone building, is to get your muscles to work against gravity. Translation: *weight-bearing exercise.*

Choosing the Ideal Weight-Bearing Exercise

Regular weight-bearing exercise in children and teenagers is a great way to produce strong bones. In adults, weight-bearing exercises help to maintain and build bone mass. For adults 65 or older, this form of physical activity can be used to reduce the rate of bone loss, avoid bone injuries by improving muscle strength, coordination and balance and if you are feeding your body what it needs, there is no reason you can't continue to feed the bones what it needs and also build bone mass even if a small amount. Determination often gets results no matter what age.

Weight-bearing aerobic activities involve doing aerobic exercise on your feet, with your bones supporting your weight. These forms of exercise work directly on the bones in your legs, hips and lower spine to slow mineral loss. Your skeleton recognizes the need for added strength and your body gets minerals to the right locations to accomplish this. If you don't use it, you lose it.

Each time your foot hits the ground, stress is applied to your bones, which respond by maintaining or increasing their strength, which can be measured in terms of increased bone mineral density. I always aim to combine several weight-bearing exercises. This makes my workout routine more exciting and I feel that I'm working all my bones and muscles when I do a variation.

Here's a simple, straightforward, thorough weight-bearing workout that is part of the Whole Body Bone Building and Body Slimming Program (call (888) 456-1597 for the whole kit with charts and exercise travel equipment) that you can do at home with minimal equipment. It includes a warmup, circuit resistance training and cardiovascular workout, cool-down, and stretches, and will take about 45 minutes to one hour of your time. The circuit resistance training (which is the magic that builds bone mineral density for strong bones) can be done 3 to 5 times a week and should only take approximately 15 minutes from start to finish so if that's all you can do-than just do that!

HOME CARDIOVASCULAR WORKOUT

Here, you boost heart rate to a place where your cardiovascular and respiratory systems (collectively, known as the cardiorespiratory system) become stronger and more efficient. Over time, your cardiorespiratory system will improve its ability to move oxygen to the muscles and to "burn" fuel in the cells to make energy, and as a result your endurance and level of exercise tolerance will rise. If you aren't an exerciser, you may be astonished at how much and how quickly your body will increase its capacity . . . before you know it, even if you don't end up leaping tall buildings with a single bound, at least, you'll have far more energy and feel stronger in your body.

Of course, begin gradually, and if you have any health condition, check in with your doctor before starting a new exercise program.

Your options here are many. You can:

- walk, jog, or run outdoors
- play basketball, tennis, or soccer
- use a treadmill or elliptical machine to do these activities indoors
- bounce on a mini-trampoline
- step up and down on a specially made step (which you can buy at a sporting goods store)
- purchase an exercise video with a cardio segment

If you are pressed for time, you can also skip the dedicated cardio segment, choosing instead to do a strength-training circuit, where you do multiple sets of strengthening exercises without stopping (more on this below). It's a true well rounded program if you can do them both though.

The goal here is to get your heart rate up to a level termed "aerobic"—i.e., that builds your cardiorespiratory fitness—and keep it there for 20 to 60 minutes. You'll want to aim for anywhere from 50 to 85 percent of the maximum heart rate for someone of your age range. Check the American Heart Association's target heart rate chart, reproduced below, to see what your goal heart rate should be. Following these guidelines will help you to get to or stay at your healthiest weight; the more cardio you do, the more calories you'll burn in your workout.

Find your pulse in your wrist or on one side of your throat, or put your palm over your heart. Since it's challenging to measure your heart rate for a full minute, you can use the 15-second count while exercising. Another alternative: invest in a heart rate monitor. If you have trouble with the whole heart rate concept, you can use the "talk test": while in your target heart rate range, you should be able to speak a complete sentence without taking a breath—but you should be good and ready for a breath by the time your sentence is complete.

AGE	TARGET HR ZONE (50–85%) IN BEATS PER MINUTE (BPM)	AVERAGE MAXIMUM HEART RATE (100%) IN BPM	TARGET HR IN BEATS PER 15 SECONDS
20–29	100–170	200	25–42
30–39	95–162	190	24–41
40–49	90–153	180	23–38
50–59	85–145	170	21–36
60–69	80–136	160	20–34
70+	75–128	150	19–32

Begin with a short warm-up—two to five minutes should be adequate—with your heart rate at or just below the low end of the recommended range for your age group. Then, increase your intensity to get into the proper range. If you're doing a shorter workout, try for the high end of the range; if you plan to do a longer workout, stay in the low end. At the end of your cardio segment, take the intensity back down a few notches again as you did with your warm-up. Then, you'll be ready for your strength-training segment.

STRENGTH-TRAINING EXERCISES

Surely, you've heard the old tale of the young boy who got a bull calf as a gift. Every day, he lifted the calf, and as the calf grew, the boy became stronger and stronger, until he was a grown man and could lift his full-grown bull. This is the fundamental concept behind strength training: lifting increasing amounts of weight to continue increasing strength.

Although you won't likely need to do any cow-wrangling or similarly heavy lifting, a reasonable strength-training program can do wonders for your physique, your bones, your balance, and your resistance against injury, no matter what your age.

To build muscle and bone strength, I recommend using free weights, weight machines, resistance bands, or water exercise (not swimming, but using water exercise props to work the muscles against the resistance of the water). You can also do exercises that use your body weight as resistance. Exercises that gently stretch your upper back help to improve posture and reduce damaging stress on your bones while maintaining bone density. Keep in mind that learning a new kind of physical activity is also good for your brain, helping to stave off age-related memory loss.

> ### CIRCUIT TRAINING: COMBINING STRENGTHENING AND CARDIO WORKOUTS
>
> Circuit training is an excellent short-cut method that allows you to combine strength training and cardiovascular work. Simply perform the recommended number of repetitions of each of the strength-training exercises described in this chapter, then go straight into the next strength-training exercise without stopping to rest. Perform all of the exercises on the circuit without stopping, then begin again. Try for three circuits, which will likely take you 20–30 minutes to complete. Check your heart rate a couple of times as you go to ensure that you're in your target range.

If you believe or already know that your bones have become weakened or brittle, certain exercises can induce injury.

If this is the case, avoid high-impact exercises such as running, jogging or jumping until you can build back nutrients in the bones and your doctor clears you for more intense exercise. These activities compress the spine and lower extremities, which can lead to fractures in weakened bones. In any workout, a person with weakened bones needs to make sure that he or she always has something to grab in the case of a loss of balance. Work with your doctor or a physical therapist to design a safe program that will build your strength and get you to where more intense exercise is safe for you.

Avoid exercises where you bend your body forward and rapidly twist your waist. Rounding your low back and then twisting your body puts unnecessary torque on weakened vertebrae. Any twisting motion with the shoulders or waist should be performed slowly, with a long exhalation, and should only be performed when the spine can be held tall and straight. This includes touching your toes, doing full twisting sit-ups, or using a rowing machine. These movements compress the bones in your spine.

Your best bet if you have osteoporosis: consult with a physical therapist to determine the best and safest exercise program for you.

Here, I've included exercises to address every major muscle group—abdominals and trunk, upper and lower back, hips and legs, and arms and shoulders—to be done with body weight and a resistance band. You can buy these bands at any sporting goods store and the "Whole Body Bone Building and Body Slimming Program" (see www.energyessentials.com) includes them with the Resistance Ball for a great bone strengthening regimen, and the best thing about them is their portability—you can bring them on vacation or to work.

The *areas most vulnerable to bone loss* include the *hips, wrist,* the *spine, forearm,* and *neck.* I've included exercises designed to strengthen these specific areas as well as a whole body well rounded program.

If you belong to a gym, invest in a session with a trainer or bring a friend who can teach you how to get a full-body strengthening workout, safely and efficiently. Most gyms also offer classes that apply resistance bands, weights, weighted bars, or body weight to work the major muscle groups.

I've given advice about breath pattern here, mainly to give you an idea of how slowly these exercises should be performed. Don't rush! Take each repetition slowly and don't let momentum take over.

You can do these in any order you like.

Even if you find yourself immobile—let's say you're ill or have broken a hip—don't take it lying down! What I mean to say is that you can always build strength and challenge your body, even if there are certain areas you can't move. Take it slow, check with your doctor but you can and should continue to challenge yourself. Strengthen your hamstrings, your quadriceps, your neck, whatever you can strengthen. Even if it's just a little bit every day, you're using the strength of your will to send the message to your body that it's still needed. No matter your age or health, exercise is hugely important in the big picture—every bit as important as nutrition. It gives you energy, helps you stay motivated and can lift even the most sour of moods. Get used to the idea that you'll be doing some kind of exercise daily until you take your last breath!

A note on resistance band usage: when you use the band to do an exercise, stretch it more or less taut to begin with so that you are pushing against resistance throughout the exercise. Adjust the band's tautness so that you can feel your muscles working, and so you're more or less worn out by the time you finish the prescribed number of repetitions—as though you probably couldn't do more than one more rep if you were to keep going.

LEG EXERCISES

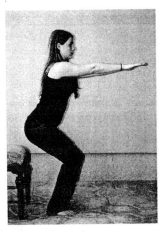

1 **Chair squats:** Place a chair behind you, then take a step away from it. Squat your hips back towards the seat of the chair, counterbalancing by reaching both arms out in front of you. Keep your heels on the floor and don't thrust your knees out past your toes. When you feel your buttocks touching the chair, don't let your weight fall into it; instead, stand back up, bringing your arms back down to your sides. Repeat 10 times, taking a long exhale as you squat your hips back and taking a full inhale as you stand back up. You can increase the intensity here by standing on your resistance band and holding it in both hands, so that you straighten your legs against resistance.

2 **Pliés:** Stand facing the back of the chair and place one or both hands on it. Start with your feet together, then lift your toes and rotate your legs outward from the hips so that the knees face outward and the feet form about a 90 degree angle. Then, maintaining the turnout in both legs, step the feet 2 ½ to 3 feet apart. Now, you're ready to begin: press the knees out and back behind you as you lower your hips toward the floor. The heels stay down; be sure not to

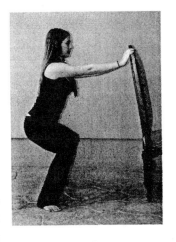

push your hips out behind you, but drop the tailbone straight down towards the floor. When you've reached your maximum stretch, straighten the knees and return to the starting position. Repeat 10 times, exhaling as you descend and inhaling as you straighten the knees.

3 **Standing lunges:** Stand with one side to the back of your chair, resting the fingertips of one hand on it for balance. Bend the knee farthest from the chair, squatting back on that leg as you press the other leg back into a long lunge, exhaling. The front knee should

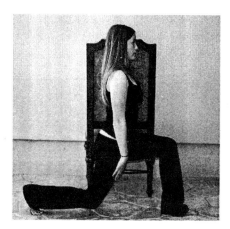

not go past the toes of that leg, and the heel of that foot should stay on the ground; aim for a 90 degree angle in that knee. Then, straighten the bent knee, inhaling, as you bring the other leg back forward to return to the starting position. Repeat 8–10 times, then turn around and lunge 8–10 times on the other leg.

4 **Heel raises:** Bring your feet together, hip-width apart. Rise onto the balls of your feet, pressing your ankles towards each other to prevent yourself from rolling onto the outsides of your feet; then lower the heels. Inhale as you rise and exhale as you drop the heels. Repeat 12–16 times. As you get stronger, you can try doing 8–10 repetitions balanced on one foot, then doing the same number of repetitions balanced on the other foot.

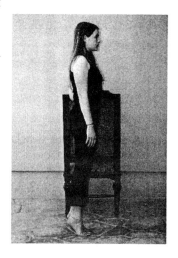

5 Quadriceps strengthener: Sit on your chair with feet flat on the floor.

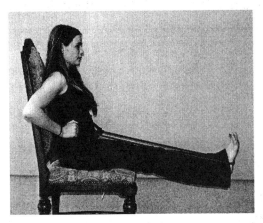

Exhaling, extend the legs all the way straight out in front of you, and inhale to return the legs to the floor. Repeat 12–16 times. As you build strength, you can use your resistance band to do one leg at a time: tie the band around both ankles as you sit, then extend one leg straight, pulling the band taut, 8–10 times; then, do the second leg.

6 Hamstring strengthener: Stand facing the back of the chair again, with feet together. Keeping the thighs and knees together, bring one heel towards the buttock on the same side, exhaling; then, inhaling, lower the foot almost to the ground. Repeat 12–16 times, then switch legs. You can use the resistance band here, too, in the same way you used it in leg exercise #4: tie it around your ankles before beginning.

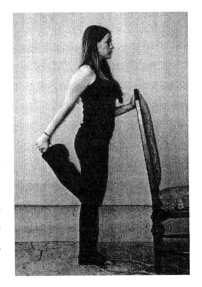

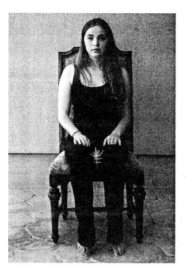

7 Inner thigh/hip strengthener: Hold a small ball between your knees while sitting at the edge of a chair. Press your knees inward, squeezing the ball, on the exhale; relax on the inhale (but not enough to drop the ball). Work up to 20–30 repetitions.

8 Outer thigh/hip strengthener: Stand with one side facing the front of a couch. Press the outside edge of the ankle against the couch as you exhale, and release on the inhale, working up to 15 on each side. You can also do this exercise with your resistance band and: knot the band around both ankles and step side to side against resistance, 20 times, or sit in a chair with legs extended and feet off of the floor, pressing the ankles away from one another on the exhale, 20–30 times.

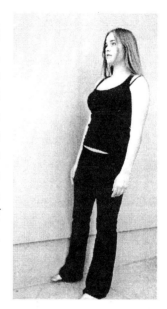

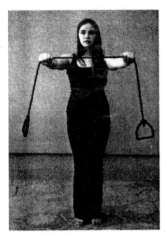

1 Lat pulldown: The *latissimus dorsi* are the muscles that attach your arms to your spine, and they are important for shoulder and trunk stability. Hold your resistance band overhead in both hands—not directly overhead, but far enough in front of you to see it in your peripheral vision when you look forward. Holding one arm steady, pull the other arm out and down towards your ribcage, drawing the band taut and stopping as your elbow nears or touches your ribs. Return to starting position and repeat 8–10 times before switching sides. Exhale as you pull down and inhale as you return to the starting position.

2 Push-ups or resistance band chest presses: Push-ups are still the best exercise for building strength in the chest, and can be adapted and modified for any fitness level. You can do wall push-ups, where you step your feet back from a wall and lean your weight into it, then do push-ups from there; or on the floor, on all fours or with the body straight but resting on the knees. If you're able to do traditional push-ups with the balls of your feet on the ground, by all means go for it! Inhale as you lower and exhale as you straighten the arms. Do as many as you can do before you feel almost totally worn out. If you would rather stay seated or standing, use your resistance band to do a chest press: loop the band around your upper back and under both arms,

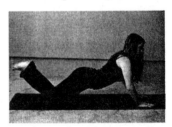

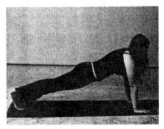

then hold an end in each hand. Lift your elbows and drop your shoulders, so that the entire arm is on a plane parallel to the floor. Press your arms straight out in front of you as you exhale, and bring your thumbs together out in front of you when arms are straight; then return to starting position as you inhale. Repeat 12–16 times.

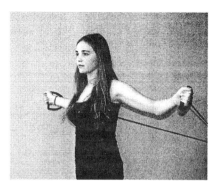

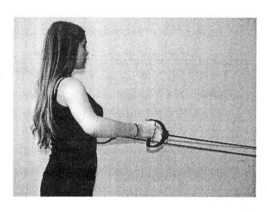

3 **Upper back rows:** You can do these seated or standing. Loop your resistance band around the leg of a heavy table or something similarly sturdy, then take one end of the band in each hand, facing the wrapping point of the band. Then, pull the band back towards you with both hands, exhaling, keeping your elbows down at your sides. Pull back as far as you can comfortably, then return to starting position. Repeat 12–16 times. You can add another set of these upper back rows with elbows lifted and shoulders dropped, arms on a parallel plane to the floor, to work a different set of upper back muscles; if you do so, perform 12–16 repetitions of that version as well. [can also do upper back fly's with hand weights, seated in a chair]

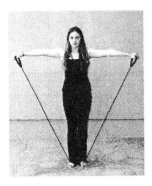

4 Shoulder raises: Stand on your resistance band with one or both feet and hold one end in each hand. With elbows slightly bent, lift the hands up towards the ceiling, stopping at shoulder height. You can lift the hands in front, to the sides, or alternating. Exhale as you lift the hands and inhale as you return the hands to their starting position.

5 Neck presses: This is a great one for people who work at desks or spend a lot of time in traffic jams or on public transportation. You can exercise your neck in all four directions, building muscle and bone strength, with this isometric exercise: put the palm of one

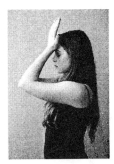
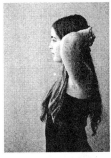
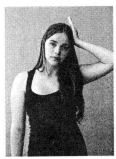
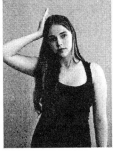

hand against your forehead and press your forehead into the palm for a slow count of five, exhaling; release and inhale on a count of two, then repeat four more times. You can also place the small ball under your chin and put pressure on the ball for resistance. Then, put one hand against the back of your head and press into the hand five times with the same rhythm. Repeat the same rhythm and number of repetitions to each side by putting one palm against the side of the head and pressing the head sideways into it, and repeating to the other side.

ABDOMINAL AND LOW BACK EXERCISES

1 **Abdominal "crunch:"** Lie on your back on a mat or carpet. Bend both knees and put the soles of both feet on the floor. Reach both

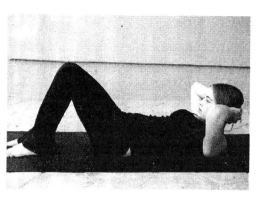

hands behind your head and interlace your fingers to support the weight of the head. Tuck your chin down towards your chest. Contract your abdominal muscles, so that you feel your belly button moving in and up the front of your spine and your low back pressing into the floor. Maintain that contraction and lift your shoulders off of the floor as you exhale and lower them on the inhale. Repeat 16–30 times.

2 **Bicycle:** Begin in the same position as in abdominal exercise #1, hands supporting the head.

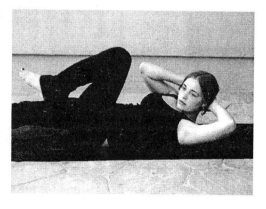

Contract your abs to lift your shoulders off of the floor. Lift your feet off the floor, knees bent at 90 degrees, until your lower legs (shins) are parallel to the floor. On an exhale, bring your right knee in and put your left foot on the floor as you cross your left elbow towards the right knee. On the inhale, return both legs and the upper body to the starting position; on the next inhale, bring the left knee in, right elbow in, right foot to the floor; exhale back to starting position. Repeat this entire sequence 10 times.

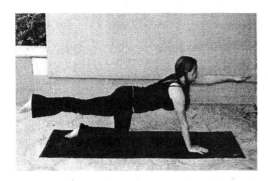

3 Low back strengthener #1: On all fours, look down at the floor. Extend your right leg out behind you and your left arm out in front of you on an exhale. Hold this posture for 4–5 breaths. Return the arm and leg to the starting position, then repeat with left leg behind and right arm extended. Repeat once more on both sides.

4 Low back strengthener #2: Lie on your belly on the floor, forehead touching the floor and hands placed palm down at shoulder level, elbows bent up into the air behind you. Extend fully through the legs, then inhale, lifting the chest off of the floor using the back muscles. Gaze out in front of yourself. You can leave the palms down on the floor or lift them up. When it comes time to exhale, lower the forehead, chest, and hands back onto the floor. As you grow stronger, you can lift the legs at the same time you lift your chest and hands.

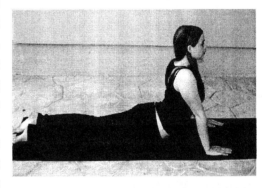

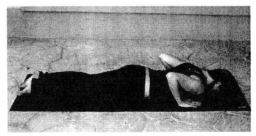

STRETCHING FUNDAMENTALS

Stretching is the *yin* to strength training's *yang*. We heat up the muscles and build strength against resistance, then lengthen and release the muscles with careful, gentle stretching. Together, these two elements of a workout program will help prevent injury and bone and joint deterioration.

Hold each of these for at least 30 seconds. Don't bounce or push hard; simply take deep breaths, pressing more deeply into the stretch as you exhale.

1 Hamstring stretch: Sit on your chair. Extend one leg straight out, foot flexed (toes pointing upwards), with the other leg bent and the sole of that foot on the floor. Interlace your fingers and lean both hands onto the thigh of the bent leg. Push your tailbone back and up towards

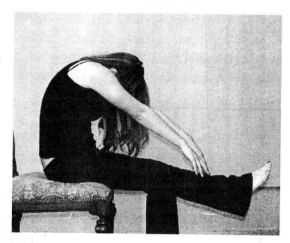

the ceiling so that your low back becomes very straight; look out in front of you. Then tilt your entire upper body forward over the extended leg. You will probably feel the stretch at the point where the back of your thigh meets your pelvis. Repeat with the other leg.

2 **Quadriceps stretch:** Stand and hold the back of your chair with one hand. Bend one knee and reach back to try to grab the foot

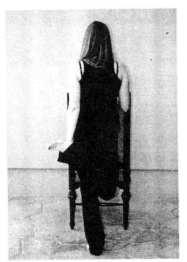

of the bent leg. If you can't reach it, use your resistance band—just loop it around your ankle and hold both ends in one hand. Then, stand tall on the standing leg and press the hip of the other leg forward until you feel a stretch in the front of the hip and thigh in the bent leg. Repeat with other leg.

3 **Calf stretch:** Stand with your toes on the edge of a step, heels hanging off; hold something for balance if necessary. Bend one knee and press the other knee straight; hold for 30 seconds, then bend the other knee and press the other knee straight for another 30 seconds.

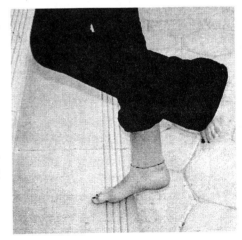

4 **Upper back stretch:** Standing or sitting, extend one arm across your chest and use the other hand to press it in and across your body. Hold for 30 seconds, then repeat with the other arm for 30 more seconds.

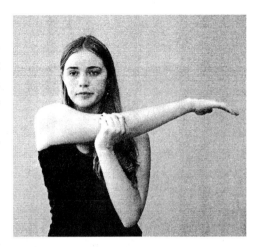

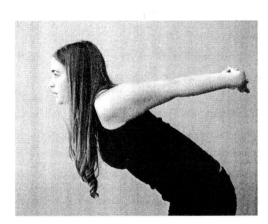

5 **Chest stretch:** Standing, clasp your hands behind your back; roll your shoulders back and down. Lift your hands up towards the ceiling.

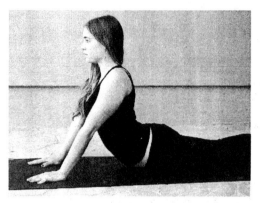

6 Abdominal stretch: Lie on your belly, head turned to one side. Place your hands next to your head, forearms on the floor, elbows tucked into your body. Press with your arms to lift your chest, lifting the top of your head towards the ceiling and arching your back gently, until you are supporting your weight on your arms, lower belly, hips, and the front of your legs. Roll your shoulders back and down and keep the back of your neck long.

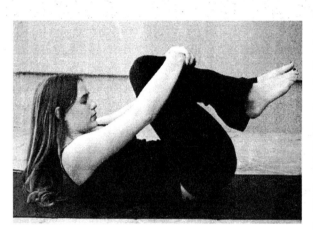

7 Low back stretch: Lie on your back on the floor and hug both knees into your chest, gently rocking your hips side to side to massage the low back. After at least 30 seconds, let both knees drop to one side, keeping both shoulders on the floor and extending your arms out shoulder-height. Stay there for 30 seconds, then switch the knees to the other side.

. . . and that's all! Congratulations—you've just done the Whole Body Building and Strengthening workout! (visit www.energyessentials.com or call (888) 456–1597 if you want the entire program with the Exercise Wall Charts, The Food and Symptom Chart, and the Exercise Band and Ball) You can do this workout every single day, or two or three times a week, alternating with or alongside long walks or other cardiovascular activities.

Find ways to be active in your everyday life: climb more stairs, do heel raises while in line at the bank, sit on an exercise ball instead of an office chair, and play with your children or grandchildren at the park instead of sitting on a bench. An hour a day of moderately intense exercise is ideal, but studies show that even 10 minutes of activity three times a day can improve strength and cardiorespiratory health.

Mix it up; find some physical activities that you enjoy. Your body was made to work, play, dance, and stretch! Once you get into the habit of exercising daily or almost daily, you'll feel so much better that you'll wonder why you waited so long.

Chapter Seven

Taking Charge of Your Family's Health

I've heard that too much information can be dangerous . . . but few will argue with the fact that little information is even *more* threatening to life and limb. Curiosity may have killed the cat, but human inquisitiveness is a necessary aspect of making good choices in our complicated modern world.

One danger of learning too much is that it can get you really ticked off. As I researched for this book, I found that the more I learned, the angrier and sadder I got. I saw plainly that industries that were specifically developed to help guide Americans to live a healthy life were actually hurting us. I found a web of deception, filled with misinformation that is making certain industries richer at the expense of Americans' health and lives.

Huge profit stands to be made even off of the illnesses that strike as a result of this misinformation. There's a lot of money to be made in "healing" people—or, more accurately, in getting them on a regimen of multiple prescription drugs for life in order to stave off illnesses that could have been avoided with the right information and guidance. Staying healthy and living a whole body bone building lifestyle may not be *easy* in a world full of comfy chairs, sedentary pursuits, hot-fudge sundaes, far too many choices regarding nutritional supplementation, and conflicting recommendations from so-called experts . . . but it isn't complicated, either. In these pages, I hope I've offered you the basic information you need to keep things simple and super-healthy.

The calcium deceptions that plague our nation today are totally outrageous. We have heeded the advice that calcium supplementation is essential, but the vast majority of calcium supplements available to us contain calcium derived from rocks, chalk and shells: sources that are completely *unidentifiable* to—and *un-absorbable* by—our bodies. In many cases, these supplements are lacking the nutrient minerals and co-factors required for our bones to use the calcium. At best, this means our bones don't benefit from the calcium horse pills we're choking down day in and day out; at worst, they may lead to mild hypercalcemia, which has in turn been associated with health problems.

There are natural, organic, inexpensive ways to supply our bodies with the calcium and nutrient co-factors we require. Companies instead turn to rocks, shells and stones that need to be crushed by machines so that they can charge the consumers a pretty penny while building their fortunes on products that cost penny's. It's ludicrous, outrageous and it must stop!

While we thought milk was once a wholesome way to fill our bodies with calcium, we now know it was never a viable way to get calcium. After years of being slammed with "Got Milk?" campaigns, I was angry to learn that the majority of milk we drink is loaded with rBGH, a hormone associated with some serious diseases. Modern engineering to make cows more efficient is backfiring; we are not only poisoning ourselves, the cows, and the environment with the practices used to produce cheap dairy. With the growing number of people being diagnosed with Crohn's disease and its increasingly obvious link to Johne's disease in cattle, why haven't we grasped the fact that this is a mad experiment that has gone awry and that it must be stopped?

I'm frustrated with manufacturer claims that do not stand up to scientific studies in terms of promoting health. I'm sick of being sick and given the *wrong* instructions on how to go about living a disease-free, healthy lifestyle.

Our Westernized, highly processed foods are making us sick.

Making efficiency and ease a priority has begun to rob too many of us of long-term health. As rates of cancer, osteoporosis, Alzheimer's disease, and heart disease continue to rise and rise, when will we see this as a clear sign that how we are taking care of ourselves is *not working?* That the foods we are eating in our fast-paced lives are creating a major acid-base imbalance that is killing us?

Our movement away from colorful fruits and vegetables is leaving our bones and bodies *starved* of the nutrients needed to thrive for a lifetime. Filling up on animal protein and bone-leaching sodas is a sure-fire way to welcome broken bones, hip fractures and serious disease.

As we discussed in Chapter Four, the warning signs are everywhere. Children are breaking more bones, women are experiencing more hip fractures, with men not far behind in this bone crisis. Red flags are being waved everyday in the headlines, but nothing is being done to slow this catastrophe. We're advised to eat more dairy and choke down more calcium carbonate horse pills—even as evidence piles up that these are not only not helping, but they may be contributing to the problem.

It's time to slow down, to take the time to protect our bodies from needless diseases and life-altering health challenges. While many nutrients are key for living a fabulous, long, healthy life, the calcium equation is especially important. If we don't feed our bones the proper forms of calcium and its co-factors, we stand defenseless against a disease expected to afflict huge numbers of people in years to come. Few maladies are as preventable with simple changes in diet, supplementation, and lifestyle. Our cardiovascular and digestive systems will also benefit from getting the calcium equation just right.

It is my hope that you are now empowered to make educated decisions for you and your family that will insure long-term bone health. Please take this information and share it with those you care about. As a single person, I can only hope I make a dent. As a group, we have a stronger voice to spread the word, to expose the deceit of the so-called experts and to protect our families from serious illness in their lifetimes.

Until now, there was no clear direction on what you could do take care of your bones and overall health. I hope this book has helped ease the confusion on what type of absorbable calcium and chaperone minerals you need to feed your bones at every stage of life.

We all deserve to lead a long, healthy, disease-free, spiritually fulfilling life. It is my goal to empower each and every one of you to weed through the deceit and get on track for a most meaningful future.

Catie Wyman-Norris

Recipes

These are some of my favorite calcium/calcium co-factor-mineral rich recipes.

CATIE'S SUPER SALMON BURGERS

Rich in calcium and other needed co-factors; makes four burgers

Ingredients:

1 (14.75 oz.) can salmon, drained and flaked
1 egg, lightly beaten
¼ cup unsweetened organic soy or almond milk
2 tbsp. finely chopped onion
1 garlic clove, minced
¼ cup minced red and yellow bell pepper
1 tsp. dried Italian seasoning blend or Herbs de Provence
¼ tsp dried Chipotle Pepper Seasoning
¼ tsp. fresh ground black pepper
1 tsp. lemon zest
¼ tsp. garlic salt
⅓ cup wheat-free pretzel crumbs
½ tbsp. chopped cilantro

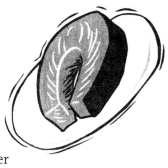

½ tsp. oregano
¼ tsp. thyme
1 tbsp. fresh virgin olive oil
4 wheat-free buns or bread

Garnishes: lettuce, tomato, avocado, onion, chile-cilantro spread (see next recipe)

Combine salmon and next 15 ingredients in a bowl. Mix well. Form mixture into 4 equal patties about ½ inch thick.

Heat oil in a stainless steel skillet over medium heat. Add patties and cook 5 minutes on each side. Top bottom halves of buns with salmon burgers. Garnish if desired. Cover with bun tops.

CATIE'S CHILI-CILANTRO MAYONNAISE SPREAD

Rich in vitamin E and antioxidant phytonutrients

Combine:

½ cup low-fat safflower mayonnaise
2 tbsp. chopped mild green chiles
2 tbsp. chopped fresh cilantro

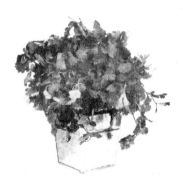

Process in a blender; pour into a small bowl with a spoon for serving.

Spread on burgers or use as a dip for sweet potato fries (see below).

BROCCOLI RABE WITH PIRI PIRI

1 large red bell pepper, roasted, peeled and
    finely chopped
1 tbsp. red wine vinegar
½ tsp. sea salt
⅛ tsp. ground black pepper
3 cloves garlic, finely chopped
1 tbsp. olive oil
6 cups (about 8 oz.) broccoli rabe
Sea salt and black pepper

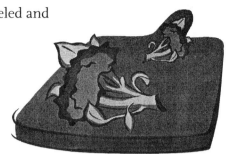

1. To make piri piri, combine red pepper, vinegar, salt, pepper and
   garlic. Refrigerate in a glass jar until needed.
2. In a large sauté pan, heat olive oil on medium heat. Trim tough
   ends from broccoli rabe and discard. Chop rabe into large
   pieces; add to pan and sprinkle with sea salt and pepper. Wilt
   for 2 minutes. Add piri piri and toss. Cook 1–2 minutes more
   and remove from heat. Taste and adjust seasoning.

CATIE'S SPLENDID SWEET POTATO FRIES

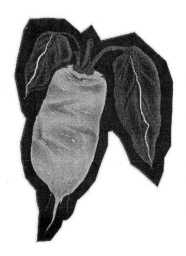

Makes four servings

Julienne two sweet potatoes. Toss
with olive oil, sprinkle with crushed
garlic and sea salt and freshly ground
black pepper. Place on a lightly
greased baking sheet and bake at 400
degrees for 20–25 minutes, turning
occasionally or until crispy and
golden brown.

CRUSTLESS VEGGIE-SPINACH QUICHE

Serves 4

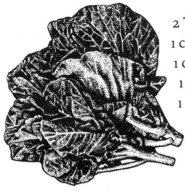

2 Tbsp. extra-virgin olive oil
1 cup white button mushrooms, sliced
1 cup red bell pepper, sliced
1 lb. shredded soy or almond cheese
1 ½ cups chopped baby bok choy
½ cup chopped spinach leaves without
stems
4 organic eggs

Preheat oven to 350°F. Heat oil in a heavy stainless steel skillet over medium-high heat. Sauté mushrooms and peppers 5–7 minutes, or until softened. Cool. Blend all ingredients together and season with salt and pepper to taste. Pour into glass buttered pie pans. Bake 40 minutes.

FLATBREAD PIZZA WITH SPINACH, BABY BOK CHOY GREENS AND CAPERS

Serves 8

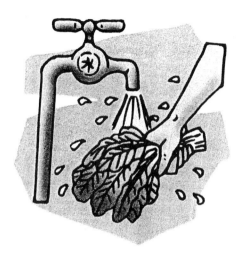

Dough
½ tsp. yeast
12 scant ounces lukewarm
  water
1 ¼ pound Bob Mills wheat-free
  baking mix (or his bread
  mix) —about 4½ lightly
  spooned and leveled cups
½ tbsp. sea salt
Olive oil

Toppings

2 medium-large onions, thinly
  sliced
2 tbsp plus 2 tsp. olive oil
12 cloves garlic
16 cherry tomatoes, halved
1 tbsp chopped fresh basil
½ tbsp. chopped fresh oregano
2 cups (about 1 oz.) spinach
  leaves, chopped
2 cups baby bok choy greens,
  chopped
3 tsp. capers, drained
½ cup freshly grated parmesan
  cheese

1. To make dough: In a mixer of food processor fitted with a dough blade, combine yeast and water and let stand for 5 minutes. In a bowl combine flour and salt; add to yeast mixture and mix for 3–4 minutes. Form into four balls. Coat with olive oil and place on a baking sheet, leaving space between them. cover with plastic and refrigerate for 1 hour or up to 2 days (dough will rise).

2. For toppings: sauté onions in 2 tablespoons oil over medium-high heat, stirring often, until brown and caramelized, 20 minutes. Set aside. Peel garlic, drizzle with a little olive oil, place on a baking sheet, and roast at 375 degrees for 10–15 minutes, turning once. Cool and chop. In a medium bowl, toss cherry tomatoes with basil, oregano and 1 teaspoon olive oil.

3. Preheat oven to 400 degrees. On a floured surface, roll out dough balls to make four thin, 9–10 inch crusts; place on baking sheets. Bake for 3 minutes. Cool slightly (leave on baking sheets). Increase over to 500 degrees. Brush each crust with ¼ teaspoon olive oil. Sprinkle with caramelized onions, then garlic, then spinach and bok choy. Top with tomato-herb mixture, capers, and soy, almond or organic cheese. Bake on middle rack for 6–8 minutes, until crusts are crispy with bubbles.

Per serving: 343 cal, 17% fat cal, 6g fat, 2g sat fat, 4mg chol, 10g protein, 61g carb, 3g fiber, 472mg sodium. Rich in plant calcium.

GUILTLESS ASPARAGUS PESTO PIZZA

Serves 4

¾ lb. asparagus, cut into ¾ inch lengths
1 Tbs. oil
1 Tbs. pine nuts
1 cup fresh basil leaves
1 clove garlic, chopped
2 Tbs. Romano or Parmesan cheese, grated
1 Tbs. oil
1 large baked cheese pizza crust, or Amy's Wheat Free Cheese
    Pizza
1 Lg. Roma Tomato, seeded and chopped
½ lb. shredded mozzarella cheese, or Shredded Soy Mozzarella
¼ cup grated Parmesan cheese

Preheat oven to 350°F. Place asparagus in a
steamer basket over boiling water. Cover pan
and steam 5 minutes, or until bright green
and almost tender. Drain, rinse under cold
water and rinse again. Spread pine nuts on
plate and toast for 3–5 minutes, until lightly
browned. Transfer pine nuts, olive oil and
next 4 ingredients to a blender or food
processor and process until smooth.
Spread pesto over crust and top with asparagus, pepper, mozzarella and Parmesan. Place pizza on an oven tray
and bake 15 minutes, or until topping
is golden brown.

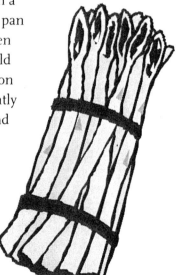

HONEY-CURRIED KALE WITH CARAMELIZED ONIONS

Serves 6

½ medium onion, thinly sliced
1 tbsp. olive oil or vegetable oil
1 tbsp. curry powder
1 tbsp. honey
1 tsp. fresh lemon juice
½ bunch kale (about 4 oz.), tough stems removed, leaves chopped
   large
(or 6 cups packed chopped kale)
2 tbsp. Braggs liquid amino acid
¼ cup water

Sauté onion in oil over medium heat until dark brown and caramelized, about 20 minutes. Stir in curry powder, honey and
lemon juice. Add kale, Bragg's, and water. Cook for 5 minutes,
tossing repeatedly until kale is chewy but tender.

Per serving: 50 cal, 42% fat cal, 3g fat, 0g sat fat, 0mg chol, 1g protein, 7g carb, 1g fiber, 209mg sodium. Rich in plant calcium.

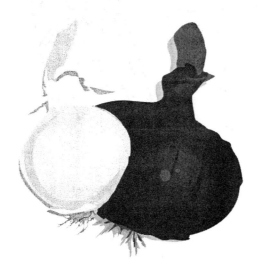

ORGANIC GREENS AND VEGETABLE SALAD WITH LIME-GINGER VINAIGRETTE

Lime-Ginger Vinaigrette (makes 2.5 cups)

4 tbsp. chopped shallot
1 ½ tbsp. chopped fresh ginger
2 tbsp. minced Serrano pepper
3 tbsp. chopped fresh cilantro
½ cup fresh lime juice
¼ cup rice wine vinegar
3 tbsp. agave nectar
4 tbsp. Bragg's Amino Acids
3 tbsp. sweet chile sauce
2 tsp. sea salt
1 tsp. ground black pepper
½ cup vegetable oil

Salad

½ pound mixed organic greens
1 cup julienned jicama
1 cup julienned carrot
1 cup julienned red bell pepper
½ cup sliced or chopped water chestnuts
½ cup fresh cilantro leaves
20 fresh mint leaves, torn if large

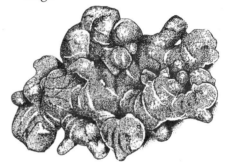

1. Combine all dressing ingredients except oil in a food processor or blender and pulse for 1 minutes. Slowly drizzle in oil and pulse to emulsify.

2. In a large salad bowl combine all greens and vegetables. Drizzle with about ¼ cup vinaigrette and toss. Taste and add more dressing if desired.

Per serving: 45 cal, 28% fat cal, 1g fat, 0g sat fat, 0mg chol, 1g protein, 8g carb, 2g fiber, 118mg sodium. Rich in plant calcium and minerals.

SPIRALS WITH BABY BOK CHOY AND FENNEL STOCK

Fennel Stock

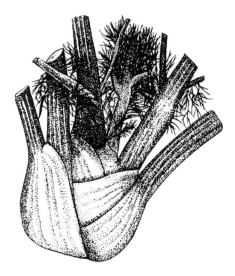

1 leek, cleaned and chopped
1 stalk celery, chopped
1 carrot, peeled and chopped
1 medium bulb fennel, chopped
¼ bunch parsley
10 whole peppercorns
3 bay leaves
8 cups water
2 tbsp. olive oil
½ pound Baby Bok Choy, chopped
1 ½ tbsp. chopped fresh garlic
1 large tomato (8 oz.) chopped
1 tsp. sea salt
½ tsp. ground white pepper

4 cups barely cooked spiral pasta or wheat free spirals (8oz. uncooked)
4 oz. goat cheese, crumbled

1. Combine all stock ingredients and bring to a boil. Reduce heat to medium and simmer until reduced to 2 cups, about 1 ½ hours. Strain, pressing to extract liquid. Discard solids.

2. In a large saucepan heat olive oil. Add bok choy, toss and wilt for 2 minutes. Add garlic and tomato and toss for 2 minutes. Add 2 cups fennel stock, salt and white pepper and bring to a boil. When boiling, add barely cooked pasta; reduce heat and toss until heated through. Add goat cheese; toss 2 minutes more. Taste and adjust seasoning. Serve in shallow bowls.

Per serving: 267 cal, 36% fat cal, 11g fat, 5g sat fat, 15mg chol, 10g protein, 33g carbs, 2g fiber, 497mg sodium. Rich in plant calcium and minerals.

FUSILLI PASTA WITH CREAMY WILD MUSHROOM SAUCE

Rich in calcium and vitamin D

Ingredients:

12 oz. wheat-free fusilli pasta
2 tbsp. olive oil
½ lb.wild mushrooms, including chanterelle and white button
   mushrooms; stems trimmed, wiped clean and thinly sliced
¼ cup chopped shallots
1 tbsp. chopped garlic
2 tsp. minced fresh thyme leaves
⅔ cup finely chopped green leaves of bok choy (an Asian cabbage)
1 tsp. sea salt
½ tsp freshly ground pepper
1–½ cup organic, unsweetened soy milk
½ cup finely grated Parmesan cheese
2 tbsp. finely chopped chives
¼ cup white wine

In a large pot of boiling salted water, cook the pasta until al dente. Drain and return to the pot. Cover to keep warm.

Meanwhile, in a large sauté pan, heat the oil over medium-high heat. Add the mushrooms and cook, stirring until soft, three to four minutes. Add the wine, shallots, garlic, thyme, bok choy, salt and pepper and cook, stirring until fragrant, about two minutes. Add the soy milk; increase heat to high and bring to a boil. Reduce the heat and simmer until the sauce thickens and reduces enough to coat the back of a spoon, about five minutes. Add the Parmesan and adjust the seasoning to taste.

Add the pasta, stir to coat with the sauce and cook until pasta is heated through, about one minute. Remove from the heat and divide among 4 serving bowls or plates. Sprinkle each serving with chives and serve immediately with a green salad. Rich in plant calcium and whole food vitamin D.

How to Cook Leafy Greens

Not sure how to cook calcium-rich greens? Here's a brief primer.

Chard and Spinach

Of course, you can eat some greens like spinach raw; chard and turnip greens aren't so great unless cooked. There are so many options here—you can throw spinach leaves into hot soups or into salads, or chop fine and add to sauces. You may want to cut the leaves from the stems if making chard; the stems can be added to the pan for two or three minutes before adding the leaves.

Wash thoroughly and chop. Put some extra-virgin olive oil or peanut oil into a frying pan; add some chopped onions or garlic if you like, then throw in the chopped greens and cook until soft. Spinach takes only a few moments to cook through, and chard, takes longer. With chard, you may want to steam for a couple of minutes by putting the lid on the pan. Add some toasted pine nuts and/or dried fruit to chard if you like. (My favorite combination: rainbow chard with golden raisins and pine nuts.)

One of my favorite ways to eat these greens is mixed into scrambled eggs. Cook the greens, then pour some scrambled eggs in right over them. Turn the heat down and flip like an omelette. A dash of tamari or Bragg's amino acid (soy but wheat free alternative) sauce can be added to the eggs before scrambling. You'll be astonished to find out how much green stuff you can pack into a couple of scrambled eggs!

Collard Greens and Kale

These greens are tougher and more bitter than chard, cabbage, or spinach. They can be cooked like chard and spinach, but require longer cooking time; best bet is to quik boil them and drain them before putting into the pan with onions and/or garlic.

Kale and collards are a good addition to soups or stews, especially those that contain beans and small amounts of smoked meat (turkey bacon, or turkey). Before adding to these foods, strip the leafy parts from the fibrous stems and chop. Allow for a good 15 minutes' cooking time if not precooked before addition to the soup or stew. My favorite is making hummus wraps with a spicey chili sauce & sprouts.

Bok Choi

Aside from the recipe for fusilli, bok choi can be prepared in many ways. It can be chopped and added to Asian-flavored soups, stir-fried in sesame oil with a dash of soy or wheat free Bragg's Amino Acids, or steamed. It's delicious with baked or broiled fish.

Calcium-Rich Dressings and Dips

Surefire ways to get bioavailable calcium into the diet of every person in your family.

Tofu Dressing

Ingredients:

½ low-fat, firm, silken tofu
3 tbsp. rice vinegar
3 tbsp. miso (made from fermented soybeans; salty and delicious!)
¼ cup water
2 tbsp chopped or minced fresh ginger (you can buy this in jars at most markets)
2 tsp. salad oil (safflower or canola)
1 clove crushed or minced garlic (also available pre-minced in jars)

Instructions:

Combine all ingredients in a blender and blend until smooth. Or, place all ingredients in a bowl and use a handblender. Add more water if needed to thin. Use as a dip for raw vegetables.

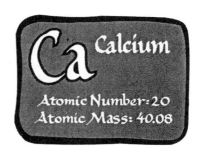

Ca Calcium
Atomic Number: 20
Atomic Mass: 40.08

ALMOND BUTTER DRESSING

Ingredients:

½ cup tofu

3 tbsp. almond butter

2 tbsp. wheat-free tamari soy sauce

4 tbsp. rice vinegar

2 tbsp. agave syrup (a more healthy substitute for sugar; can be
found in most health-food stores; can substitute honey or
brown rice syrup)

1 ½ tbsp. fresh ginger, peeled, chopped or minced

4 tbsp. coconut milk

1 chopped scallion

Instructions:

Combine all ingredients in
blender and puree, or use
handblender in bowl. Use
as a sauce for noodles, over
chicken or cooked vegeta-
bles, or as a dip.

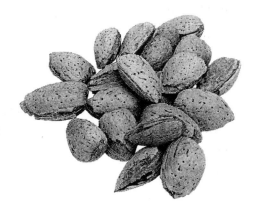

References

Abraham GE, Grewal H, "A total dietary program emphasizing magnesium instead of calcium. Effect on the mineral density of calcaneous bone in postmenopausal women on hormone therapy," J Reprod Med 1990 May;35(5):503–7.

Cedar Sinai Hospital Physician's Case Study: (L. Ory. 2008) www.energy essentials.com for full report.

Al-Delaimy WK, et al, "Magnesium intake and risk of coronary heart disease among men," J Am Coll Nutr 2004 Feb;23(1):63–70.

Associated Press, "Light-zapped mushrooms filled with vitamin D," April 18, 2006, http://www.msnbc.msn.com/id/12370708/; accessed April 9, 2008.

Bede O, et al, "Urinary magnesium excretion in asthmatic children receiving magnesium supplements: a randomized, placebo-controlled, double-blind study," Magnes Res 2003 Dec;16(4): 262–70.

Biser-Rohrbaugh A, Hadley-Miller N, "Vitamin D deficiency in breast-fed toddlers," J of Pediatr Orthaped 2001;21:508–11.

Brody J, "Drink your milk: a refrain for all ages, now more than ever." NYTimes.com/2003/01/07/science/07BROD.html

Brown C, (2001). "Kids breaking more bones." Gotmilk.com

Brown, SE, "Are your bones running on empty?" Ladies Home Journal 2005; 35–39

Chan JM, et al, "Dairy products, calcium and prostate cancer risk in the Physicians' Health Study." Am J. Clin Nutr 2001; Oct;74(4):549–54.

Dawson-Hughes B, Harris SS, "Calcium intake influences the association of protein intake with rates of bone loss in elderly men and women," *Am J Clin Nutr* 2002 Apr;75(4):773–9.

DeLuca HF and Zierold C, "Mechanisms and functions of vitamin D," Nutr Rev 1998;56:S4–10.

Dunford R, et al, "Chemical oxidation and DNA damage catalyzed by inorganic sunscreen ingredients," FEBS Lett 1997 Nov 24;418(1–2):87–90.

Ebert R, Jakob F, "Selenium deficiency as a putative risk factor for osteoporosis," International Congress Series, Nutritional Aspects of Osteoporosis, March 2007:158–64.

Feskanich D., et al, "Milk, dietary calcium and bone fractures in women: a 12 year prospective study." Am J Public Health 1997; Jun;87(6):992–7.

Firoz M, Graber M, "Bioavailability of US commercial magnesium preparations," Magnes Res 2001 Dec;14(4):257–62.

Grinspoon S, E. Thomas, S. Pitts, E. Gross et al. Prevalence and Predictive Factors for Regional Osteopenia in Women with Anorexia Nervosa. Ann Intern Med 133(10): 790–794 (Nov 2000).

Guthrie Catherine, "Why Magnesium Matters," Alternative Medicine 2003 Sept:43.

Hamilton Kirk, "Pain (Musculoskeletal) and Hypovitaminosis D," Clinical Pearls "One-Liners," April 2004, Vol, 3, No.4: 15–16.

Hayes CE, Hashold FE, Spach KM, Pederson LB, "The immunological functions of the vitamin D endocrine system," Cell Mol Biol 2003; 49:277–300.

Hazelrigg SR, et al, "The efficacy of supplemental magnesium in reducing atrial fibrillation after coronary artery bypass graft," Ann Thorac Surg 2004 Mar;77(3):824–30.

Heaney RP, "Long-latency deficiency disease: insights from calcium and vitamin D," Am J Clin Nutr 2003;78:912–9

Hemphill, RR, "Hypercalcemia." www.emedicine.com/emerg/topic260.htm, 2006.

Holick MF, "Evolution and function of vitamin D," Recent Results Cancer Res 2003;164:3–28.

Holick MF, "Vitamin D: the underappreciated D-lightful hormone that is important for skeletal and cellular health," Curr Opin Endocrinol Diabetes 2002;9:87–98.

Kahan Z., et al. (2006). "Elevated levels of circulating insulin-like growth factor-1, IGF-binding globulin-3 and testosterone predict hormone-dependent breast cancer in postmenopausal women: a case-control study." Int J Oncol Jul;29(1):193–200.

Karjalainen J, et al, "A bovine albumin peptide as possible trigger of insulin-dependent diabetes mellitus," New England Journal of Medicine 1992;327:302–7.

Landau R, Scott JA, Smiley RM, "Magnesium-induced vasodilation in the dorsal hand vein," BJOG 2004 May;11(5):446–51.

LeBoff MS, Kohlmeier L, Hurwitz S, Franklin J, Wright J, Glowacki J, "Occult vitamin D deficiency in postmenopausal US women with acute hip fracture," J Am Med Assoc 1999;251:1505–11.

Lo CW, Paris PW, Clemens TL, Nolan J, Holick MF, "Vitamin D absorption in healthy subjects and in patients with intestinal malabsorption syndromes," Am J Clin Nutr 1985;42:644–49.

Lukert BP and Raisz LG, "Glucocorticoid-induced osteoporosis: Pathogenesis and management," Annals of Internal Medicine 1990;112:352–64.

Ma DF, et al, "Soy isoflavone intake increases bone mineral density in the spine of menopausal women: meta-analysis of randomized controlled trials," Clin Nutr 2008 Feb; 27(1):57–64.

Maier JA, et al, "Low magnesium promotes endothelial cell dysfunction: implications for atherosclerosis, inflammation and thrombosis," Biochim Biophys Acta 2004 May 24;1689(1):13–21.

Martinez ME and Willett WC, "Calcium, vitamin D, and colorectal cancer: a review of the epidemiologic evidence," Cancer Epidemiol Biomark Prev 1998;7:163–68.

Michon P, "Level of total and ionized magnesium fraction based on biochemical analysis of blood and hair and effect of supplemental magnesium (SlowMag B6) on selected parameters in hypertension of patients treated with various groups of drugs," Ann Acad Med Stetin 2002;48:85–97.

Naghii MR and Samman S, "The role of boron in nutrition and metabolism," Progress in Food and Nutrition Science 1993; 17(4): 331–349.

Need AG, Morris HA, Horowitz M, Nordin C, "Effects of skin thickness, age, body fat, and sunlight on serum 25–hydroxyvitamin D," Am J Clin Nutr 1993;58:882–5.

Nielsen FH, et al, "Effect of dietary boron on mineral, estrogen, and testosterone metabolism in postmenopausal women," FASEB J 1987;394–7.)

No authors listed, "Vitamin D," http://ods.od.nih.gov/factsheets/vitamind.asp

No authors listed, "International scientific committee warns of serious risks of breast and prostate cancer from Monsanto's Hormonal Milk," Cancer Prevention Coalition 2003.

No authors listed, "Oral magnesium successfully relieves premenstrual mood changes," Obstet Gynecol 1991;78(2):177–81.

No authors listed, "Starbucks milk not doing a body good," CNN.com, 2007.

Norton A, "Plant estrogens may fight menopausal bone loss." Reutershealth. com, 2004.

Patrick L, "Comparative absorption of calcium sources and calcium citrate malate for the prevention of osteoporosis." Altern Med Rev 1999; 4(2): 75–85.

Rodriguez-Martinez MA and Garcia-Cohen EC, "Role of Ca2+and vitamin D in the prevention and treatment of osteoporosis," Pharmacology & Therapeutics 2002;93:37–49.

Scanu AM, et al, "Mycobacterium avium subspecies paratuberculosis infection in cases of irritable bowel syndrome and comparison with Crohn's disease and Johne's disease: common neural and immune pathogenicities," J Clin Microbiol. 2007 Dec;45(12):3883–90. Epub 2007 Oct 3.

Schechter M, "Does magnesium have a role in the treatment of patients with coronary artery disease?" Am J Cardiovasc Drugs 2003;3(4):231–9.

Scott FW, "Cow milk and insulin-dependent diabetes mellitus: is there a relationship?" American Journal of Clinical Nutrition 1990;51:489–91.

Sojka JE, Weaver CM, "Magnesium supplements and osteoporosis," Nutr Rev 1995 Mar;53(3):71–4.

Stendig-Lindberg G, et al, "Experimentally induced prolonged magnesium deficiency causes osteoporosis in the rat," Eur J Intern Med 2004 Apr;15(2):97–107.

Touyz RM, "Magnesium in clinical medicine," Frontiers in Bioscience 2004 May 1;9:1278–93.

Vaarala O, Paronen J, Otonkoski T, Akerblom H K, "Cow milk feeding induces antibodies to insulin in children—A link between cow milk and Insulin-Dependent Diabetes Mellitus?" Scand J Immunol 47:131–135, 1998.]

van den Berg H, "Bioavailability of vitamin D," Eur J Clin Nutr 1997;51 Suppl 1:S76–9.

Vieth R, "Vitamin D supplementation, 25–hydroxyvitamin D concentrations, and safety," Am J Clin Nutr 1999;69:842–56.

Weaver, J. (2006). "Can stress actually be good for you?" MSNBC.com.

Webb AR, Pilbeam C, Hanafin N, Holick MF, "An evaluation of the relative contributions of exposure to sunlight and of diet to the circulating concentrations of 25–hydroxyvitamin D in an elderly nursing home population in Boston," Am J Clin Nutr 1990;51:1075–81.

Weikert C, et al, "The relation between dietary protein, calcium and bone health in women: results from the EPIC Potsdam cohort." Ann Nutr Metab 2005;49(5):312–8.

Weng FL, et al, "Risk factors for low serum 25–hydroxyvitamin D concentrations in otherwise healthy children and adolescents," American Journal of Clinical Nutrition, July 2007, Volume 86, Number 1, Pages 150–158.)

REFERENCES: The Whole Body Bone Building Program:

www.energyessentials.com
www.curesinthekitchen.com
Whole Food Supplements:
www.energyessentials.com (888) 456–1597
www.radiantgreens.com (818) 591–9355
Whole Food-Non Isolated Hemp Protein:
www.energyessentials.com (888) 591–9355
Andrew Keech, PhD
(480) 710 6770

Plant Iron:
Floradix (check your local health food store)
Catie's Whole Food Plant Iron
(888) 456–1597
Pomegranate with 40% Elegiac Acid:
www.radiantgreens.com or (818) 591–9355
Whole Food Vitamin C
www.energyessentials.com
(888) 456–1597

BIOLOGICAL DENTISTRY
Ezekiel N. Lagos, D.D.S.
www.biologicaldent.com

STEM CELL THERAPY REFERENCE:
Healing Bones, Joints & Tissue with your own stem cells
Dr. David Steenblock, D.O.
Personalized Regenerative Medicine
26381 Crown Valley Parkway, Suite 130
Mission Viejo, CA
(800) 300–1063

HOPE4CANCER INSTITUTE
Dr. Tony Jimenez, M.D.
482 W. Ysidro Blvd. # 1589
San Ysidro, CA 92173
(619) 468–9209
www.hope4cancer.com

OPERATION SMILE REFERENCE:
Join Humanitarian, Actress Roma Downey & Producer Mark Burnett to
    help children with Cleft Palate
www.onesmile.org

BOOK REFERENCES:

"DEADLY HARVEST"
The intimate relationship between our health and our food.
Geoff Bond

"Miracle Super Foods That Heal"
The power of greens foods in healing and rejuvenation.
"Miracle Red Super Foods That Heal"
The power of red foods in healing and rejuvenation.
"Miracle Detox Secrets"
Incorporating detoxification into your lifestyle naturally.
    Plus pH balancing.
Tony O'Donnell, N.D., C.N.C.
www.radiantgreens.com

"Going Back To The Basics of Human Health"
Avoiding the fads, the trends and the bold faced lies.
Mary Frost, M.A.
"Magnetic Miracles"
Using magnets for radiant health.

"The Truth About Vitamin C"
The most important antioxidant for your health.
Overcoming Our Two Top Killers!
Catie J. Norris
www.energyessentials.com

TELEVISION SHOW REFERENCES:
"The Cures in the Kitchen"
www.curesinthekitchen.com

The Green Channel
Check your local listings
HEALTH WEBSITES:
www.radiantgreens.com
www.energyessentials.com
www.awakenings.com

Index